P9-CRS-079

INFORMED CONSENT

Books by John A. Byrne

The Whiz Kids

Odyssey (coauthored with John Sculley)

The Headhunters

INFORMED CONSENT

JOHN A. BYRNE

McGraw-Hill
New York   San Francisco   Washington, D.C.   Auckland   Bogotá
Caracas   Lisbon   London   Madrid   Mexico City   Milan
Montreal   New Delhi   San Juan   Singapore
Sydney   Tokyo   Toronto

Library of Congress catalog card number: 95-80169

McGraw-Hill

A Division of The **McGraw·Hill** Companies

1 2 3 4 5 6 7 8 9 0   DOH/DOH   9 0 0 9 8 7 6 5

ISBN 0-07-009625-2

McGraw-Hill books are available at special quantity discounts to
use as premiums and sales promotions, or for use in corporate
training programs. For more information, please write to the
Director of Special Sales, McGraw-Hill, 11 West 19th Street, New
York, NY 10011. Or contact your local bookstore.

This book is printed on acid-free paper.

Informed Consent: A medical doctrine based on the notion that every patient has a right to decide what's going to be done to his or her body. It requires doctors to inform patients of all the risks and benefits connected with an operation or procedure. Patients must not only be informed of such risks, they also must fully understand them.

CONTENTS

"This above all: to thine own self be true,
and it must follow, as the night the day,
Thou canst not then be false to any man."

—*Shakespeare*

PROLOGUE

Precisely four weeks earlier, Colleen Swanson had been out cold on an operating table at Mount Sinai Hospital in Cleveland. The gowned surgeon had labored for three hours to remove a pair of silicone breast implants that had been in her chest for 17 years. Colleen wanted the plastic bags taken out of her body because she was convinced they were the cause of health problems that had severely eroded her life for years.

Since the grueling operation, she had been bandaged from her collarbone to her waist. Today, on a bright and beautiful summer morning in July of 1991, she would get the first glimpse of herself without the silicone implants that had been a part of her for so long. Colleen's husband, John, had already left home for his job at Dow Corning Corporation—the company that had manufactured the implants. He was one of those steady-and-sure managers and had once loved his job and his life in little Midland, Michigan, the quintessential company town. But for years now, John Swanson had shared his wife's anguish and distress. He had comforted her through a series of mysterious ailments that ranged from severe migraines to debilitating joint pain and extreme fatigue. And when he came to believe, as Colleen did, that his company's product was destroying his wife, John Swanson supported her decision to have the implants removed.

But today, in the privacy of their home, Colleen wanted to face the consequence of that decision on her own. She had purposely failed to remind her husband that it was the day for her to remove the bandages. "I really felt I wanted to deal with it myself," she recalls. So Swanson had left to drive the 10 miles to Dow Corning's headquarters, not knowing that

Colleen was about to experience one of the most ghastly moments of her life.

Ever since her surgery, she had wondered again and again what she would look like. A petite and gracious woman of 55, Colleen was always impeccably turned out. Her hair, her clothes, and her demeanor reflected her conservative Midwestern background—quiet taste and a demure sense of tradition. She had sought the implants only to bring her small, uneven breasts closer to average and to make her clothes fit better. She had been assured that few, if any, risks went along with her new look.

Now, she wondered if her husband would be able to make love to her again. Would everything return to normal? Would she despise her appearance? "I had all kinds of ideas of what I might look like," she says. "I only knew one thing for sure: that I wouldn't look anything like the way I had been. I knew it was going to be bad because my surgeon had told me that most of my breast tissue had been destroyed." No amount of preparation, however, could sufficiently fortify Colleen for what she was about to see.

She spent hours that morning just trying to summon the courage to do what the surgeon had suggested. She drew a warm bath and eased herself into the tub, gently splashing water over the bandages. She hoped that the water would pen-etrate the clear plastic tape and lessen the pain of its removal. But the bath failed to loosen the dressing, and finally Colleen gave up.

Later in the afternoon, around 2 P.M., she tried again. Alone in the master bedroom on the second floor of their Williamsburg colonial home, the wife of the Dow Corning executive lowered the shades. She slipped off her blouse and blue jeans and quietly lay down on the bed. She began to pull at the tape that held the white gauze bandages in place. She started at the top left, peeling the cover from her body, gritting her teeth against the pain.

Only when the bandages were completely removed and tossed aside did Colleen, still lying on the bed, glance down at what was left of her breasts. She didn't want to take it all in at once. At best, she hoped to see some semblance of roundness, some reminder of the adult female that she had been 17 years before. But what she glimpsed made her cry out, then shut her eyes, not wanting to see anymore.

She climbed out of bed and walked slowly to the adjoining bathroom, consciously avoiding the full-length mirror on the bedroom wall. Instead, she went to the smaller mirror above the sink. Before flicking on the light, she closed her eyes once more and tensed. Finally, she stared at her reflection. What she saw overwhelmed her with anguish and tears.

Six-inch scars, pinkish red because they had not yet completely healed, curved across each half of her chest where the creases beneath her breasts had once been. The lesions—about a quarter of an inch thick—stretched around to the sides of her upper body. All of her chest—ravaged and sore—was framed as if it were a picture by the raw outline of the sticky tape that had held the bandages to her body for four weeks.

Where her breasts had been, there were now just slight ridges of folded, discolored skin—like deflated balloons that had held air for a long time. The wrinkled skin supported nothing. The left side of her chest, where more silicone had apparently leaked into her body, was nearly concave. Her nipples were inverted, caved into her chest because there was no longer any breast tissue left to support them.

Colleen stared at herself for four or five minutes, grieving the loss of her breasts. She didn't recognize the person in the mirror, the frightened and pitiful woman whose trembling body was forever disfigured.

Finally, she stepped into the shower and let the water stream over her body, washing the yellowish seepage and dried blood from the wound. She tried to calm herself and relax, but she couldn't hold back the sobbing. "I cried and cried and cried," she remembers. "I cried for a long time."

CORPORATE RECUSAL

Everything he did that morning, he did slowly, deliberately, briefly postponing what would be an irreversible decision in his career. It was September 18, 1991, and John E. Swanson was about to tell Dow Corning Corporation, his employer of 26 years, that he could no longer accept its decision to continue selling silicone breast implants. Not when thousands of women were complaining of serious health problems because of them. Not when his own wife had finally come to believe that her agonizing descent into one illness after another had been caused by the implants he had told her were safe 17 years earlier. And certainly not after his wife had endured the painful removal of the implants—she would be disfigured for the rest of her life.

Swanson, the guardian of Dow Corning's much-admired ethics program, would go into recusal. A funny word, seldom heard in corporate corridors, possibly never heard before at Dow Corning, recusal meant that he would have nothing to do with the Dow Corning product that had been stitched into the chests of more than 1 million women since 1963. It meant that the 56-year-old manager, who had once helped promote the devices and had even helped draft a defense of them for *Ms.* magazine, would refuse to discuss implants, create memos about them, or help the company defend itself against the growing onslaught of criticism.

To some, Swanson will appear a sympathetic and unlikely hero in a monumental corporate tragedy. To others, he may seem little more than a turncoat, or, as one Dow Corning executive calls him, "an odd duck" who refused to play the game. But the story he lived is emblematic of the ethical and moral conflicts that can face any manager or executive. At one time or another, anyone may find himself or herself in strong ethical disagreement with an employer. What happens when personal values clash with corporate beliefs? What happens when you make a moral choice that separates you from the company's official position and from your colleagues in a close-knit organization? What happens when long-established trust between you and your company deteriorates? Should you compromise your sense of right and wrong? Or should you risk your job, your career, and your standing in the community by declaring that you'll have no part of what you believe to be a corporate misdeed? Swanson, concerned though he was about the possible consequences of his stand, was about to make the break that would provide answers to those difficult questions.

It was a break that would tear apart every aspect of his professional and personal life. And all of it—his career, his friendships—mattered tremendously to Swanson. He was not an oddball, a gadfly, or a manager disgruntled by a poor performance review. Earnest and cautious, he had an unblemished record as manager of corporate internal and business communications. So trusted was Swanson that he had counseled three Dow Corning chief executives on a wide variety of internal and external communications issues and had often written their speeches and presentations. For more than a decade, he had been active in semi-annual area operating board meetings that brought together the company's 40 top executives from around the world. Swanson was a respected conservative, a country club Republican in Midland, Michigan, a law-abiding, God-fearing town. And as the only permanent member of Dow Corning's Business Conduct Committee, he had earned a reputation for ethical probity within and outside the company.

Swanson had created, overseen, and sustained a highly respected ethics program that had been the subject of three Harvard Business School case studies. And unlike many other companies, Dow Corning had put teeth into its ethics initiatives. The company's code of ethics wasn't just another bland, sound-alike statement reminiscent of the Boy Scout oath. It didn't end up in the back of an employee handbook for all to ignore or forget. The code was mailed to each employee at home with a letter from the chief executive. It was translated into seven languages and hung in offices, hallways, and lobbies of Dow Corning buildings around the world. It was reprinted in company publications, flashed on screens during management presentations, recited during face-to-face compliance reviews. Swanson was its guardian. As the company's former chairman, Jack Ludington, once put it: "John's leadership in the area of business conduct has helped to give Dow Corning a distinguished reputation in this area and is an example to other corporations worldwide." Indeed, John Swanson was as close as you could get to the conscience of his corporation.

He not only acted the part, he looked it as well, a throwback to the Organization Man of the fifties. Lean and fairskinned, with light blue eyes, closely-cropped dark hair, and an expressive face, Swanson looks as though he was made to sit behind an executive's desk in a prudent Brooks Brothers suit. He boasts all the attributes you might expect in a Midwesterner of his generation: He is responsible, loyal, sober, and discreet. He can be witty, but not wildly so. Even the way he speaks, in a mild and smooth voice like that of an announcer on some middle-of-the-road radio station, breeds confidence.

Swanson's personal and professional lives, as was inevitable in little Midland, were closely bound. Their circle of casual friends was composed of people he worked with, though he maintained close friendships with several couples who did not work for either Dow Corning or Dow Chemical. Still, they socialized together at dinner parties and company events. An avid golfer, Swanson spent Saturdays playing with a diehard group of golfing colleagues who traversed the state to play a variety of challenging courses. One of Swanson's good Dow Corning friends—his golfing partner in the Midland Country Club's annual invitational tournament—was Dan Hayes, who in 1985 became president and chief executive of the Dow Corning subsidiary that made the implants.

So it was all the more shocking that it was John Swanson who brought the crisis home to Dow Corning's corporate headquarters in Midland. Questions about the safety of silicone implants had been getting greater attention from both Congress and the Food and Drug Administration. A growing number of women, alleging that they had developed a variety of ailments, including crippling immune-system diseases, as a consequence of the implants, were filing lawsuits against Dow Corning. A highly vocal consumer group in Washington was lobbying the FDA to take action. And the media were just beginning to turn on the pressure. News reports told how the company had applied a full-court press to prevent damaging memos and studies from reaching the public. Even the local newspaper, the *Midland Daily News,* generally an unabashed supporter of the company, had begun to criticize Dow Corning, calling it secretive and slow to respond to the rising tide of complaints. Though Dow Corning's executives tried to play down the crisis, treating it as little more than a battle with the press, the outcry would eventually threaten the company's viability. All this because of a product that accounted for less than one percent of Dow Corning's $2 billion in revenues and, according to the company, was not profitable.

Few executives inside the company realized how vulnerable Dow Corning would become. But Swanson had known almost instinctively that the controversy had the potential to overwhelm the company and destroy its public image. To Swanson, the company's executives seemed willfully unresponsive—to the government, to the media, and especially to the women with legitimate complaints. Swanson, of course, didn't know whether or not silicone leaking from a breast implant could cause debilitating and potentially fatal autoimmune diseases such as rheumatoid arthritis and scleroderma. He had no idea if silicone could cause a person's immune system to attack the body's connective tissue, as some alleged. After all, he was not a scientist or a chemist. He wasn't familiar with all the laboratory tests. But for him, the allegations about silicone's dangers were almost beside the point. Swanson believed that the public's growing perception of a problem made it in the company's best interests to acknowledge those concerns. Even if the clinical trials and research tests eventually proved silicone to be safe, Swanson felt that by failing to heed the complaints of women with implants and refusing to act in a timely fashion, his company had behaved unethically throughout its period of involvement with the product.

Yet what Swanson did not know was far more incriminating than what he did know at the time. As the crisis enveloped the company, it had become hard for him to distinguish between truth and rumor, fact and fiction. Many of the facts were inaccessible to him, lodged deep in files in other departments and buildings. So he could hardly parcel out individual culpability or assign blame. He was not yet aware of the numerous memos penned by the company's own marketing executives and salesmen that warned of serious problems with breast implants. He had no knowledge of the document in which a marketing manager reported that, when addressing a group of plastic surgeons, he had "assured them, with crossed fingers, that Dow Corning had an active study (of safety issues) under way." Swanson hadn't heard about a memo from a company salesman relaying complaints from a "downright indignant" plastic surgeon who said Dow Corning's implants were "greasy" and had "excessive gel bleed." To put "a questionable lot of mammaries on the market is inexcusable," the salesman had written. "It has to rank right up there with the Pinto gas tank." Nor had Swanson seen any of the many letters of complaint from a prominent Las Vegas plastic surgeon who reported that he had removed ruptured implants from patients and warned that the silicone leaking from them could cause "severe body reactions" including multiple cysts. And he was unaware of the memo written by his good friend, Dan Hayes, referring to a "cover-up."

Dow Corning would play down these memos when it finally made them public. The company would argue that its marketing manager's reference to "crossed fingers" meant that he hoped the company would continue to build on its already extensive safety studies. It would say that the letters from a few of its sales representatives overdramatized isolated incidents and that concerns about gel bleeding through the product had more to do with aesthetics than performance or effectiveness.

From what little he did know, however, Swanson believed that his company had failed to prove that silicone breast implants were safe before selling them to surgeons for implantation in hundreds of thousands of women. He believed the company had failed to promptly follow up on studies that showed that silicone might cause severe health problems. He concluded that the company had failed to fully apprise women of the known risks of its breast implants so that they could make genuinely informed decisions. In his view, the company had underestimated and downplayed the complication rates for breast implants and had subsequently tried to deny any wrongdoing. Swanson believed that some managers had tried to keep the facts about problems with the product from not only the public, but also from the senior management of the company.

These were all violations of the corporate code of ethics that Swanson had spent most of his career at Dow Corning promoting. Somehow, it seemed, the company had lost its moral compass. Dow Corning, thought Swanson, was failing to live up to its own rhetoric, its own professed standards of right and wrong. Truth was not being served. Indeed, it was being left behind. It even crossed Swanson's mind that growing media scrutiny of the implant crisis would undermine the career he envisioned for himself when his days at Dow Corning were over—as an advocate of strong corporate ethics programs. Who would take him seriously once the company he worked for was widely attacked for its failure to properly test a product destined to be put into the human body?

For months, he had been brooding over the decision to recuse himself and its possible consequences. He might lose his job, or worse, become a pariah in the community to which he had devoted the better part of his life. Midland, after all, was the silicone capital of the world and fully supported its hometown Fortune 500 company. But Swanson could no longer live with the secret that, even as he worked as an executive at Dow Corning, his wife had been diagnosed as having silicone-related diseases. The fact that he had assured her at the onset that the implants were safe on what he considered impeccable authority added a grim edge to their ordeal.

Swanson had watched his wife's mystifying physical decline for years, never considering that her implants could be the cause. At first, she had suffered dreadful migraine headaches, lower back problems, numbness in both arms and hands. She would become so tired at the end of the day that she would climb into bed before dark. Then her breasts had become rock hard, and she felt a constant burning in her chest. In time, nearly unbearable pain began to sear through her left arm and hand, down into her ring and index fingers. It spread to her hips and neck. From time to time, periodic rashes would break out over her upper body, rendering her chest as red and shiny as a severe sunburn. Her illnesses, each growing into the next like an endless series of waves lapping a beach, extracted a devastating cost, eroding her energy and her life. At one point, her weight had dwindled to 89 pounds. The once perky and attractive woman John Swanson had married was a mere shadow of herself. She seemed to be dying.

Colleen Swanson had been examined by countless medical doctors—a gynecologist, an internist, a rheumatologist, urologists, a cardiovascular specialist, and an orthopedic surgeon— as well as by physical therapists. They had put her through dozens of tests, searching for everything from uterine cancer to carpal tunnel syndrome, but they could never identify the cause of her problems. Then, finally, the Swansons' own daughter had seen several women with similar symptoms on an afternoon TV talk show in late 1990. All of them had silicone breast implants, too. She called her mother from California with the news, and suddenly a light went on. It all made sense to Colleen, who had never had health problems before her implants. Initially, Swanson had refused to accept the possibility that implants made by his company could be destroying his wife's health. But slowly, as the couple sought the advice of still more doctors, he came to believe that the Dow Corning implants were the source of her anguish. The doctors had exhausted all conventional tests. There seemed to be nothing left but the possibility that her problems were caused by silicone implants.

Still, that wasn't the only reason John Swanson would ask to be removed from any work even remotely connected to the product. He was undergoing a crisis of conscience. Quietly using his position within the company to get the issue of implant safety out in the open without revealing his personal involvement was no longer bearable. He had challenged the more upbeat statements made by several executives, including his friends, on the safety of breast implants. When Dow Corning's corporate medical director charged that a top executive had ordered the destruction of internal memos that undermined the company's claims that few women with implants suffered complications, Swanson had launched an investigation. He had prodded management to suspend the manufacture and sale of implants until the mounting questions about their safety could be answered, and he had attempted to get the issue before the board of directors. But in every instance, he had been stymied. The company continued to strenuously defend the product. Swanson concluded that the medical director's charges were swept under the corporate rug. And the board made the colossal moral and public relations blunder of continuing to manufacture and sell breast implants.

Of course, John Swanson could have quit in protest. Why didn't he go public, blow the whistle? Because he had none of the damaging memos or safety tests that would hurt the company in the courtroom. He also had no hard scientific evidence to show that silicone was unsafe. Even Colleen's doctors, who had treated hundreds of silicone patients, lacked indisputable scientific documentation. They knew through experience with implanted women that common patterns of illness were appearing over and over, but they had no long-term epidemiological studies to prove that silicone caused health problems. Neither did Dow Corning Corporation at the time.

In addition, Swanson was only a few years from retirement and he was not in conflict with the company on any other issue. He had, in fact, a strongly positive overall attitude toward Dow Corning. On this issue, however, Swanson could carry the burden no longer. He was ready to cross the line, no matter what the personal cost. "The company was set in its position and it wasn't going to change," says Swanson. "Once my own position was known, the lines would be more sharply drawn, because then I would really become an avowed dissident. I would put myself out on the end of the limb. Instead of being the person who doesn't think the company is doing the right thing, now I'm the person who clearly says 'I can no longer be a part of this. And by the way, my spouse is a part of it in the most negative way.'"

He and his wife had been discussing this decision to recuse himself for weeks, and Colleen had promised to support whatever position Swanson would eventually take. "I trusted his judgment," says Colleen. "Only he knew what he was going through. We talked about how hard it was for him, but the decision was his to make. I didn't think he should quit because it would prove nothing, and neither John or I had done anything wrong."

The moment had come. Swanson entered an elevator on the first floor of DC-2, one of four square concrete buildings that rise above the cornfields of central Michigan to form Dow Corning's corporate campus. It was just after lunch, around 1:15 P.M. Stepping off on the fourth floor, Swanson went directly to the office of J. Kermit Campbell, a group vice-president who was managing the implant crisis for the company. Among the cadre of former chemists who comprised Dow Corning's management ranks, Campbell was one of the most approachable. While Chief Executive Lawrence A. Reed had a facade as cold and sterile as the pre-cast concrete at the headquarters complex, Campbell came across as caring and affable. He had a good sense of humor and a ready smile, and he enjoyed opera and good conversation. He encouraged people to call him by his nickname, Kerm.

Swanson had worked with Campbell for many years, and

he had served with him in the early 1980s on the business conduct committee. The two had traveled the world together, from Europe to the Pacific Rim. Though the Swansons had never socialized with Campbell and his wife, they had been together several times at company events. Both Campbell and Swanson were featured members of the Dow Corning Speakers Bureau, an effort by the company to reach out to the community by providing local schools, clubs, and other organizations with free speakers. Campbell's topic was "Education: A Commitment Today for Tomorrow," while Swanson spoke on "Creating an Environment for Ethical Decision Making." Moreover, Swanson suspected that Campbell might share some of his concerns about silicone breast implants. Three months earlier, Swanson had spoken privately with Campbell, urging him to suspend the manufacture and sale of implants, and Campbell had at least seemed empathetic.

Campbell's office, like all offices at Dow Corning, was sparse and open, separated from its neighbors only by movable partitions. His bookshelves displayed an eclectic collection of reading matter, from books dispensing management advice to books on language arts. A poster advertising a production of *Othello* in Midland hung on one wall. Campbell quickly waved Swanson inside, and the two seated themselves at a conference table. Kerm poured coffee from an insulated carafe.

They shared a few polite laughs over the pranks of a mutual friend, and then Swanson began what would become a long monologue. There was no easy way to start. So he simply began with his wife, describing her long illness and what they believed to be the cause. Campbell listened attentively, often nodding his head, something he did almost involuntarily.

"Kerm, I feel it's my responsibility to let the corporation know that Colleen had implants and experienced a lot of trouble," Swanson said. "She's been examined by people who are very knowledgeable in treating silicone cases."

"Locally?" asked Campbell, visibly shaken by the conversation.

"Not here," Swanson told him. "We don't have that expertise in Midland. But her providers are well experienced. She has been diagnosed with a silicone disease and had her implants removed in June."

"How is she?" asked Campbell, looking grim.

"She hasn't fully recovered. But she's very happy she had them removed and is working hard to recover and turn her life around. Still, it's been a devastating experience. She is literally without breasts. We're both dealing with that, and it hasn't been easy."

Campbell's demeanor was almost always upbeat, his countenance nearly cherubic. But as he absorbed Swanson's story his brow furled and a troubled look crossed his face. Swanson had never seen him look so morose.

"John," said Campbell, leaning across the table, "I have to tell you that Colleen is the only person I know personally who has had problems with our implants."

At the time, Swanson interpreted Campbell's statement as being his peculiar way of saying that Colleen's case was a rarity, but later he would regard it as incredible. Here was Campbell, trying to lead the corporation out of a crisis that had severely damaged its reputation and would eventually bring it to bankruptcy. Yet he had never met even one of the thousands of women who were alleging that Dow Corning's silicone had made them ill! To Swanson, it was a sure sign of just how removed from the personal side of the breast implant controversy Dow Corning's management was.

Swanson then asked to be recused from anything having to do with the implant issue. "Look," he said, "I have to distance myself from this because I don't believe the company's doing the right thing. I can't in good conscience interpret and help communicate management's views on implants to the employees. I simply cannot go through the motions anymore."

Swanson told Campbell that he thought the company's decision to conceal documents that showed Dow Corning might have known of the dangers of implants long ago was unethical, as was its defense of the product. "It was a bad business decision for the company to take its stand at the expense of a growing number of angry women and the increasingly blood-thirsty media," he said.

Campbell, Swanson thought, was accommodating and sympathetic.

"I very quickly understood his dilemma," recalls Campbell, who left Dow Corning at the height of the controversy in early 1992 to become chief executive of Herman Miller Company. "It was an untenable position to be in, to represent the company on one hand and yet have to deal with a personal crisis on the other. I never had any reason to doubt his integrity or ethics."

At the time, Campbell told Swanson, "I'll do all I can to make sure that the management of the company understands that you're not to be involved in any aspect of the breast implant issue."

The meeting with Campbell lasted several hours. By the time it was over, Swanson felt that at least one burden had been lifted from him. Conflicted for months, at times seemingly torn between his job and his wife, he had finally gotten the job responsibility and the personal ethics issue out in the open. He had no idea what would come next. Would he be fired? Would he become a corporate outcast? Would his friends and colleagues pull away from him? Perhaps, but at least Dow Corning now knew where he stood.

So Swanson would have no further involvement with the issue of implant safety at work. At home, however, he would become completely consumed by it. He would search frantically, not only for solutions to his wife's health problems, but also for explanations for his company's unethical behavior. Many evenings, after work, he would spend hours in his study, trying to make sense of it all. He had a computer research run showing abstracts of several studies and articles on silicone breast implants. He asked friends across the country to clip and send him articles on the subject from local newspapers and magazines. And he began tracing his own knowledge of and involvement with implants. He started compiling a chronology of dates and events, covering the origins of silicone breast implants and the emerging crisis. He sometimes stayed awake until the early hours of the morning, sorting through the materials and noting his reactions in the margins in neat small script.

Swanson's research was augmented by the avalanche of media coverage devoted to the breast implant controversy. Within three months of his recusal, a California woman with Dow Corning implants who suffered severe joint aches, muscle pain, fatigue, and weight loss won a $7.3 million judgment against the company that would be upheld on appeal. In early January 1992, the Food and Drug Administration would call for a 45-day moratorium on all sales of silicone breast implants. Damaging news reports—largely based on documents once sealed in numerous court cases—would charge that the company's safety studies had been inadequate and that serious questions raised by its own research and by doctors' complaints had not been answered. Finally, on April 16, 1992, the FDA would determine that adequate data to demonstrate the safety and effectiveness of silicone breast implants did not exist and would ban their use. Thousands of women, including Swanson's wife, would file lawsuits against Dow Corning, leading the company to file for federal bankruptcy protection on May 15, 1995.

The controversy and crisis are likely to plague the company for many years. Questions are now being raised about the company's other silicone medical products, from jaw replacements to penile implants. Many observers believe that a $4.23 billion accord to settle most of the claims brought by implant victims against Dow Corning and other makers of silicone breast implants will collapse. Even though it is the largest product-liability settlement in history, a federal judge has found that Dow Corning is significantly underfunded to handle the 410,000 claims that have been filed by women with implants. Moreover, thousands of other women are still pursuing their own lawsuits against Dow Corning—a circumstance that forced the company to take a pre-tax writeoff of $241 million in January 1995.

And all this time, John Swanson has meticulously tracked every development. Small incidents, nearly forgotten over the course of his long career at Dow Corning, have resurfaced and taken on great significance. These were scattered events, but they have served to erode all of his remaining confidence in his employer. Swanson recalls, for example, how in the late 1960s he attended a convention in Chicago to help introduce a new silicone product for cleaning hands. On the evening before the launch, he had received an urgent call from a Dow Corning product manager in Midland. The promotion was being called off. Apparently, the product hadn't passed the company's safety tests. "The monkey's balls shrank," the product manager told a startled Swanson. At the time, Swanson hadn't thought much of the incident. But now it troubled him. Why, he wondered, had Dow Corning decided to launch a product before the results of more extensive safety tests were in? And if silicone was inert, how could it have had that effect on a monkey? Or a human being?

John Swanson heard his colleagues and his company maintain that silicone was safe, but he began to ask himself these and many other questions for which there were no easy answers. Over the next few years, as he took early retirement and moved to another state, he accumulated huge files of publicly released corporate memos, press clippings, and court documents—anything and everything that shed even a modicum of light on what had gone wrong. What he discovered about the company he had once regarded as an exemplary corporate citizen—both highly ethical and morally responsible—shocked and disappointed him.

A COMPANY TOWN

Like most of the people who live in Midland, Michigan, John Swanson was drawn to the place because of its corporate benefactors: Dow Chemical Company and its half-owned affiliate company, Dow Corning Corporation. They are two magnanimous gods who watch over this small town in central Michigan, a two-hour drive north of Detroit. Together, they directly or indirectly employ nearly 80 percent of the population and pay nearly a third of the property taxes. Without them, there would be few reasons to live in this rather isolated town of 38,800 people.

Everywhere in Midland, a place as flat and featureless as a Formica tabletop, there is evidence of their presence and influence. The 30-square-mile area that makes up Midland is a peculiar melange of industry and suburbia, towering smokestacks and immaculate homes, chain-link fences and manicured lawns. For all the tree-lined roads that wind through residential neighborhoods, there is also the ugly maze of above-ground pipes that carry chemicals for long city blocks. The pipes wander through huge gray tanks and corrugated buildings that occupy hundreds of acres of industrial wasteland, mainly on the town's south end. Surrounding woodlands boast prominent "No Trespassing" signs with "Dow Corning" printed in white letters on a black rectangle with a bar of teal blue underneath—the corporate colors.

When the concrete blocks of factory disappear from view, residents are still reminded of corporate power and largesse. There's the Dow Gardens, an award-winning horticultural display, and the H. H. Dow Historical Museum, a collection of three timber-framed structures in which young Herbert H.

Dow, founder of the Dow Chemical empire, perfected his revolutionary process of extracting bromine from the area's subterranean brine deposits. The Grace A. Dow Memorial Library, named after Herbert's wife, occupies a campus-like setting adjacent to Midland's Center for the Arts, with its 1500-seat auditorium and three art galleries—yet another beneficiary of Dow's paternalism. The company has built or helped to build the county courthouse, the library, a community center, schools, churches, a golf course, and much more. Over the years, Dow money transformed what was once a run-down, worked-out lumbering town with 14 saloons into a pleasant and livable community with modern, up-to-date services.

The corporate gods of Midland also involve themselves in the social rhythms of the town. Each year, Dow Corning invites grammar school students to enter a Christmas card contest created by and named for Shailer Bass, a former chairman. Until recently, all the artistic submissions had to relate to a biblical theme, a requirement that drew mild criticism. The winning entries are displayed on the wall of the Center for the Arts, and the company hosts a banquet for up to 300 guests at which a Dow Corning executive hands out scholarship awards to the winning artists. Every January, the company sponsors a professional tennis tournament in town.

Yet, there seems to be something contrived about Midland. On the surface, it looks like Ira Levin's haunted Stepford, a place of happy families and pretty homes, a low-crime haven where the wives, schooled in golf, tennis, and flower arranging, seem content and compliant, attractive and undemanding. The only blacks who live in Midland are professionals or chemists—usually married. There are few black singles, and they find it nearly impossible to meet others in the area. "It's a clean town with lots of trees and beautiful gardens," says Nancy Britton, the wife of a one-time newspaper editor who spent eight years in Midland. "But the women often feel that they've stepped into the Stepford Wives syndrome. Dow and Dow Corning have a lot of power and it's used very cleverly."

Gordon C. Britton's former employer, the *Midland Daily*

News, often fails to cover the routine stuff on the police blotter, from arrests for vandalism to drunken driving. If the son or daughter of a Dow or Dow Corning executive were charged with drunken driving, you would more likely read about it in *The Bay City Times* or *The Saginaw News,* the newspapers of the two nearby cities that, along with Midland, make up what locals call the Tri-Cities. Says Britton, "Whenever I wrote critically of Dow or Dow Corning, the articles were very carefully worded. Not because anyone ever threatened me or made life uncomfortable for me, but because I recognized the sheer dominance of those corporations in the community. It's an atmosphere that says that anything that big or dominant has to be treated very carefully."

It surprised no one that when Dow Corning celebrated its fiftieth anniversary in 1993, the *Midland Daily News* commemorated the event with a special 14-page section filled with upbeat features and congratulatory advertisements from the town's merchants and suppliers. The newspaper managed to come up with more than a dozen Dow Corning stories, detailing the $157.5 million payroll the company pumped into the region's economy and the $7.5 million in property taxes it paid to Midland, while barely touching on the breast implant crisis that would eventually bankrupt the company.

The landscape isn't the only thing in Midland that is flat. Most of the buildings are squat, one-story structures—the result of a prohibition on multistory buildings that prevailed until the late 1960s, when Dow Chemical constructed its lavish corporate headquarters, known as the Pink Palace. One of the town's few noncorporate distinctions is an oddity erected in the early 1980s. Called The Tridge, it's a three-legged wooden footbridge that spans the confluence of the Tittabawassee and Chippewa rivers, where the first white settlers came to trade with the Indians. The Tridge—unique to Midland—is near the almost barren downtown, a string of empty storefronts. When the implant crisis hit, one irreverent reporter jokingly suggested that the city of Midland show its support for Dow Corning by adding two more hills to the park at The Tridge. A shopping mall on the northside of town has siphoned off most of the retail business from the downtown area since it opened in 1992. Over the past several years, a renovation project intended to beautify and add commercial appeal to Main Street has been underway. Yet even on the most beautiful Saturday afternoons, hardly anyone ventures out on the sidewalks. Instead, people are at the strips of fast-food joints and convenience stores scattered around the town that belie the community's affluence.

Young people often complain that there's nothing to do. So do visitors. "There was no more boring place in the world to work," says Arnold Zenker, a Boston-based communications consultant, who in the 1980s often traveled to Midland to work with Dow Corning executives. "I would arrange the day so when I finished up work, I could take a jog through the cornfields, eat dinner and go straight to bed." When a visiting New York journalist described Midland a few years ago as a "bleak and aging town," the *Midland Daily News* quickly conducted a telephone poll to find out if the residents agreed. By a margin of nearly two to one, Midland's own agreed with the outsider's assessment. In the winter, the days grow exceedingly cold and damp, and a bleak, gun-metal grayness falls over the city. People go for days without a glimpse of the sun.

For years the only place anyone could buy a decent meal was at the prestigious Midland Country Club, which also houses an upstairs private "Dow Club," exclusively for Dow Chemical executives. A private elevator whisks the executives and their guests to these cloistered second-floor quarters, where the drinks are more generous than those served in the downstairs bar used by the other country club members. The club building—a contemporary structure with a flat roof completed in 1931—was designed by Alden Dow, the son of the founder of Dow Chemical who had studied under Frank Lloyd Wright and impractically brought his style of architecture to Midland. Dispersed around the town are low-profiled, strikingly modern homes with aesthetically pleasing flat roofs designed by Alden Dow. But Michigan winters are tough on flat roofs, making leaks and water stains a common occurrence.

Although the country club offers ambitious managers a chance to mingle with the already anointed executives at both companies, even Midland's unusually large number of churches—58 at last count—reflect a neat hierarchical order. Many of the top-tier executives of both Dow Chemical and Dow Corning belong to either the richly endowed Memorial Presbyterian Church on Ashman Street or the First United Methodist Church on Main Street. The latter was the place of worship of former Dow Corning CEO Jack Ludington, who once served as its chairman of trustees. Both churches are stately monuments in a largely Protestant community, smart places for young up-and-comers to be seen. The most achievement-oriented wives often involve themselves in church activities with the spouses of high-ranking executives, hoping to establish social relationships that might lend their husbands a slight advantage at work.

Midland has adopted many of the peculiarities of its two Fortune 500 companies, especially Dow Chemical. The town and the two corporations are so thoroughly intertwined that each has shaped the others, reinforcing the others' strengths—and magnifying the others' flaws. If its corporate headquarters had been in New York or Chicago, Dow Corning would have been a dramatically different company. As it is, the company mirrors Midland: This workplace of Ph.D. chemists, researchers, and scientists is highly conservative and unemotional. At the same time, the fact that both Dow Corning and Dow Chemical are in the chemical industry means that the population of Midland is far more homogeneous than that of virtually any other city.

In this somewhat cloistered environment, Dow Chemical has always loomed larger than Dow Corning, and not just because of its size. Perhaps it's because Dow Chemical survived a succession of controversies over such toxic products as napalm, Agent Orange, and dioxin. The disasters raised the company's public profile and maturity. More worldly and more aggressive, Dow Chemical has long seemed eager to manage its local image. Traditionally, before selecting a new chief executive, the company would invite the community leaders to meet him for cocktails at the Midland Country Club. Dow Corning, by contrast, would simply announce the news in a press release. Recalls Britton: "The Dow Corning people were much more standoffish. Dow Corning had the attitude that if it ignored a problem, it would go away."

That aloof attitude seems to be reflected in Dow Corning's corporate headquarters' campus, which stands isolated, just outside Midland. The complex, dubbed Dow Corning Center, is on a level, 276-acre site in Williams Township. After outgrowing its Midland offices in the late 1960s, the company began moving operations to what was once farmland. Now, some 1200 of Dow Corning's roughly 8000 employees work in the six-building center.

Viewed from U.S. Highway 10, the complex, fronted by a rectangle of dancing water fountains, looks like a modern version of Stonehenge. Out of a flat, open field rise huge concrete blocks with little narrow windows. They might have been dropped from the sky. Architects used pre-cast concrete as the primary building material, a site manager once explained, to convey Dow Corning's conservatism. And so it does. Colleen Swanson says the collection of cold, sterile gray blocks always made her think of a mental institution.

With the exception of the administration building, which was named for Amory Houghton, Sr., the late chairman and long-time Dow Corning director, none of the buildings are named. Instead, they bear identifying numbers: DC-1, DC-2, and so on. DC-1, a three-story inverted pyramid, serves as the world headquarters building, and all of the company's most senior executives are located there. DC-2 holds the administrative offices for most United States operations. DC-3, the health and environmental sciences laboratory, once housed a crematorium to dispose of the dogs, monkeys, rabbits, and rats sacrificed in silicone experiments and studies carried out in the labs. DC-4, the newest of the gray edifices, is the research and development center. Underground tunnels—long gray concrete passageways—link all the buildings, making it unnecessary for anyone ever to go outside.

Inside, under the steady hum of a machine that masks the

sound of conversation—white noise, they call it—the company's employees work in an ambience of ferns, flat carpets, and modular furniture. The surroundings reflect the corporate culture, which has a low tolerance for mavericks and a high acceptance for bright people, blandly dressed and linear in their thinking. It is a place of brains and ambition, a place where people want to do well at their work and gain the respect of their peers.

Within both Dow and Dow Corning, the chemists are clearly the Brahmins. They are the miracle workers and inventors whose wizardry allows both companies to commercialize their products. Executives on the frontier of science routinely climb the corporate ladder faster than managers with any other background, to such a degree that many nonchemists believe they merely provide support. Chemists' achievements are openly celebrated at Dow Corning, with something akin to a hall of fame. One long passageway that connects two buildings is lined with 14-by-20-inch photographic portraits of chemists, with a summary of the individual's contribution under each one. At Dow Corning, greatness is reflected in those pictures on the wall.

It is the people in those portraits—and the men and women who want to be in them—who make sure the school budgets in Midland are rarely defeated. Because the chemists and professionals at Dow Chemical and Dow Corning understand the importance and value of a good education, Midland boasts an outstanding school system for a town of its size, so self-sufficient it takes no state funding.

Yet Midland's distance from any city of substance means a lack of many artistic attractions and cultural diversity. At the same time, it keeps Midland comfortably isolated from the harsher aspects of life. As a Dow Chemical president once told the local Rotary Club, Midland is "a little too provincial, a little too willing to let the world go by." At Dow Corning, the corporate culture is not just insular; it also reflects a sort of inferiority complex. When Jack Ludington became the company's chief executive officer in 1975, he sought with some success to emulate the more cosmopolitan leaders across the street at Dow. During the first week of every August, he gathered the company's top 35 to 40 executives for three-to-four-day meetings that featured lavish banquets and outside speakers. He typically dispatched Dow Corning's corporate jet, a Falcon 10, to pick up and deliver to Midland the likes of Alexander Haig, Henry Kissinger, Tom Peters, John Gardner, and others, not thinking twice about paying speakers' fees as high as $25,000 for little more than an hour's chat to 40 managers in the Round Room at DC-1. Ludington would get so carried away with these events that he would personally decide where each manager would sit, moving the names of his executives on a chart kept by his secretary as if they were bishops and rooks on a chessboard.

And when, in 1986, Dow Corning hit the billion dollar sales mark, Ludington commemorated the event by giving every employee—some 7800—a small Steuben glass American Eagle that, even though it was made by parent Corning, still cost the company $125 each. At the time, it was the largest order for a single piece of Steubenware in Corning's history. All the image-building and spending, however, failed to prevent Dow Chemical executives from privately calling the company "the little candy store across the street" —a reference to its small size compared to its nearby parent, Dow Chemical, which boasts revenues nearly 10 times those of its offspring.

For many of Midland's residents, of course, the struggle of a company to remove itself from the shadow of a parent is of little concern. More critical to them is how those two companies have shaped the culture of the community, creating social norms and attitudes vastly different from those of other cities and towns. In Midland, social acceptance has as much to do with what you are as with who you are. "If you're not a chemist or an engineer, I don't think you're ever really accepted there," believes editor Britton. "People are friendly and nice, but you're not really considered a part of the community if you don't have a science background. I was there eight years, and I still felt like a tourist."

When Colleen Swanson moved to Midland in 1973 after

marrying John Swanson, she initially found the town "cold and cliqueish." Though she eventually would forge lasting friendships with people in town, it was at first difficult to assimilate and make meaningful friends. And always, she sensed the pressure of the conservatism in this small town where everyone seemed to know everyone else's business. "Midland is a town where you do not let your hair down, because everybody is watching," Colleen says. "Protocol is very important there. There are a lot of social climbers in Midland, people who seem to spend a lot of time trying to impress others."

*   *   *

It wasn't the same in Petoskey, an old and quaint resort town that stretched along the Little Traverse Bay in northern Michigan, where Colleen had spent most of her life. Petoskey was a small town, to be sure, but it had long enjoyed a reputation as a fashionable place where wealthy Midwesterners routinely spent their summers at cottages on nearby lakes. Unlike Midland, Petoskey maintained a charming downtown area of Victorian brick storefronts—enough to make the town, with its lakefront parks, rivers, and waterfalls, something of a tourist spot on Lake Michigan.

Every year, as the weather warmed, Colleen would see the character of her hometown change with the influx of outsiders who escaped Detroit, Chicago, and other cities for the quiet comfort of Petoskey. It was not as if she had much in common with these wealthy visitors. The middle child between two brothers, she came from a family of modest means. Her mother managed a dress shop on Mitchell Street, the main drag in Petoskey, while her father worked as a carpenter. "My dad's work was very seasonal when I grew up," she recalls, "so many times in the winter he didn't have work. He would do odd jobs."

To help out, Colleen began working at the age of 11, taking care of children and ironing. At 14, she had three jobs.

She would routinely get up in the morning to get the neighbor's child off to school, serve food in the school cafeteria during lunch, and work in the kitchen of Little Traverse Hospital from 4 to 8 P.M. Frequently, she would babysit after that. Her family rarely took vacations—except to go camping and deer hunting in the local woods—and she never traveled outside the U.S., much less Michigan, before her first marriage.

At Petoskey High School, Colleen was a cute, outgoing young woman who rooted for the local football and basketball teams and danced in the school's gym on many Friday evenings. Most Sunday nights, she and her friends would chip in 50 cents apiece for gas, pile into a car and drive to the town of Walloon Lake, where Ernest Hemingway had spent each of his first 18 summers at his family's cottage. Walloon Lake, only nine miles south of Petoskey, was the place to go rollerskating at the Marsh Inn, or to ride horses through meandering trails.

Colleen was horseback riding at Walloon Lake when she met a local boy who would become her first husband. He was then 17, 2 years older than she. He lived in East Jordan, another small community 20 miles from Petoskey. He took Colleen to her senior prom and married her after a 2-year courtship, when Colleen was just 17 herself. They moved to Grand Rapids, where Bob worked for the telephone company as a splicer, and Colleen sold baby clothes and accessories at the local Kresge's.

Within a year, she had her first child, a boy they named Kelly, and two months later, her husband was transferred to Petoskey. In their second year of marriage in 1959, she gave birth to a premature daughter who died. In their third year, Colleen had another daughter, Kathy. She quickly and comfortably settled into the role of caring mother and housewife. After a stint at the Petoskey Beauty Academy, she earned extra income for her family by doing nails and facials and styling hair at Christy's Beauty Salon on Elizabeth Street, where the gossips would volunteer all the private details of their lives in a small town.

In Petoskey, Colleen Swanson had roots. She had been

born in the town and lived there for the first 33 of her first 34 years. She knew almost everyone worth knowing in town. She began her first marriage in Petoskey and ended it there 17 years later. She met John Swanson there, at the local Holiday Inn, when he and his Dow Corning colleagues came to play one of the town's golf courses. In Petoskey, she not only knew the friends of her children well, she could take comfort in knowing their parents and grandparents too. Midland was only a few hours away by car, but when she moved there in 1973, "it was a whole new ballgame for me," she says.

*   *   *

Years before meeting Colleen, however, John Swanson found Midland with its little candy store, an inviting place. He arrived in 1966, and almost immediately, like nearly everyone else who moves to the community, he suffered culture shock. An ambitious 30-year-old, married and the father of a year-old child, Swanson was moving from a big, open, and sophisticated city, Minneapolis.

The job he was taking at Dow Corning, however, was one of those career opportunities you don't turn down. The company had placed a want ad for an advertising supervisor in a national trade magazine. Swanson already boasted more than six years' experience in sales promotion and advertising, but he had worked in small, relatively unknown companies. This was a chance to work for a profitable, fast-growing corporation with operations emerging in almost every corner of the world.

He was a strong candidate for the position. After graduating from the University of Minnesota in 1959 with a degree in communications, Swanson had joined the Minneapolis Gas Company, a gas utility for the greater Minneapolis area, to work in sales promotion. The country was in a mild economic downturn at the time, and there were more than 50 candidates for the single opening at the gas company. A year later, he had switched to the local RCA-Whirlpool distributor, which supplied the gas company with appliances. Swanson had been hired as assistant manager for advertising and sales promotion. After accepting the job, he learned that he would assume his boss's job as soon as he was trained and his boss was fired. It was one of his first lessons in practical business ethics as well as a first taste of how harsh a life in business could be. However, he knew this job would be an interim stop. In 1962, Swanson had left to become manager of advertising for Fremont Industries Incorporated, a privately owned, regional manufacturer of specialty chemicals. Within two years, he had been named executive vice-president and general manager. But Fremont was a small company, with fewer than 60 employees, and Swanson, in the number two job, felt he had nowhere else to go.

Dow Corning offered much more promise. A joint venture of Dow Chemical and Corning, New York–based Corning Glass Works, it had racked up 21 consecutive years of revenue growth since being founded in 1943 in the midst of a raging world war. The venture had affiliates in England, France, Germany, Canada, Mexico, Brazil, Argentina, Australia, and Japan. At a time when science and technology seemed to promise solutions to virtually every problem faced by humankind, Dow Corning was one of the nation's corporate pioneers in harnessing science to create unique and useful products. The company boasted more than 1000 patent applications.

The foundation of its success was an unusual synthetic compound, silicone, derived from quartz and sand. For the researchers and scientists at Dow Corning, this plastic-like substance had taken on a magical dimension. Silicone was stronger than plastic, yet more flexible than glass. It was amazingly stable over a broad temperature range, from −100 degrees to 900 degrees Fahrenheit. It didn't react with many substances. And—most everyone inside and outside Dow Corning believed—silicone was biologically inert. In time, that belief would lead the company to use it in a host of medical products for the human body, from a silicone shunt for draining dangerous fluids from the skull, to silicone implants used to enlarge women's breasts or reconstruct breasts lost to cancer.

It was a wonder substance. *Fortune* magazine in 1947

devoted 11 full pages to silicone, predicting that within a decade it would be among the most important industrial plastics and synthetics. Dow Corning's first silicone product was a grease-like compound used to seal the ignition systems of Allied aircraft in World War II. After the war, Dow Corning turned silicones into products to clean eyeglasses, waterproof leather, seal buildings, and caulk bathtubs. It also came up with Silly Putty, the result of a failed 1940s laboratory effort to create a rubber compound.

To Swanson, married to first wife Grace, and father to Sarah, Midland appeared as perfect a community to raise children as any. He liked the corporate-sponsored amenities, the well-funded library and gardens, and the superb school system. So in 1966 he joined Dow Corning as advertising supervisor in a communications department of some 30 people. He worked hard and he worked long—55 to 60 hours a week. Had he been home more, he might have been more aware of the white chemical residue attached to everything in his home—a constant reminder that he lived near one of the largest chemical facilities in the world and that it regularly released pollutants into the air. Within three years, Swanson was named manager of industrial marketing with a staff of a dozen employees. He got his first real break when he wrote a successful speech for a marketing vice-president. William C. Goggin, chairman and chief executive, noticed him and began to rely on him to write his speeches and other materials. The two developed a close working relationship as Goggin began to confide in Swanson and seek his advice on issues, from establishing a Washington lobbying operation to launching an advertising campaign to clear up the confusion between Dow Corning and its two parent companies.

An autocratic executive who joined Dow Corning from Dow Chemical a year after Swanson's arrival, Goggin found himself leading the company through a wrenching reorganization. While Dow Corning was comfortably profitable, competitors were just beginning to challenge its dominance of the silicone industry. The company's employees, however, could see no immediate reason to change and were not buying into the massive overhaul. Goggin asked Swanson what he could do to gain more internal support for the major changes involved. Swanson suggested that an article in the prestigious *Harvard Business Review* might provide outside validation of the new structure—a complicated matrix of geographic areas, individual business profit centers, and specific functions. It also would be good publicity for both Goggin and Dow Corning. Swanson penned a 12-page essay filled with managerial buzzwords and organizational charts that appeared in a 1974 issue of the *Review* under Goggin's name. The article, "How the Multidimensional Structure Works at Dow Corning," soon became one of the *Review*'s most heavily reprinted features, and Goggin found himself in demand as a guru on the topic of matrix management, a trend then sweeping the corporate world.

After Goggin retired as president and chief executive in 1975, his successor, Jack S. Ludington, soon came to rely on Swanson as well. Dow Corning was becoming an increasingly global corporation, with 45 percent of its nearly $300 million in revenues derived overseas. Ludington, the first and only chief executive of Dow Corning to be born and raised in Midland, had never held a job outside the United States. Not surprisingly, he wanted to know more about how his company did business in far-flung outposts.

Among the questions that preoccupied him was whether Dow Corning adhered to the same values and principles in Europe, Asia, and elsewhere as it did in Midland, Michigan. Ludington and Dow Corning were hardly alone in their concern over corporate standards to guide the behavior of their executives overseas. Public confidence in U.S. institutions had been severely eroded in the mid-1970s by disclosures that several U.S. corporations had bribed foreign officials to gain important contracts abroad and that many executives had knowingly made illegal contributions to President Richard M. Nixon's re-election campaign. Though Dow Corning had not been involved in these controversies, it had a rapidly growing business in developing countries, where kickbacks, payoffs, and bribes were often common practices.

In May of 1976, with the blessing of Dow Corning's board

of directors, Ludington asked Swanson and three other Dow Corning managers to form the company's first business-conduct committee. The group was to learn more about how the company operated outside the United States, draft guidelines for ethical conduct, develop a workable process for monitoring business practices, and recommend ways to correct questionable activities as they became known.

Few would consider corporate ethics a riveting subject, and in 1976 Swanson was not among them. But he initially viewed the assignment as something that would pass, the product of a corporate fad that might last a year or two. He knew that, for many companies, ethics programs were mere window dressing. They published sound-alike codes of conduct suggestive of the Boy Scout oath: Employees were to be loyal, law-abiding, honest, and trustworthy. The self-serving, even pious, documents would often end up in the back of employee handbooks and soon be forgotten.

Swanson considered himself more pragmatic than idealistic. He had been keenly interested in philosophy in his college years, eagerly absorbing the teachings of such thinkers as Immanuel Kant and Sören Kierkegaard. He had spent much time thinking about good and evil, or what was moral or not, in his student years. But in a business environment, Swanson saw little application for what he considered to be abstract theories. He had been raised a strict Methodist by his family, but he never fully embraced the church's religious tenets. Yet Swanson prided himself on his integrity, one of the core values that he shared with his father, a conservative Republican who owned a family grocery store on 25th Street and 27th Avenue in Minneapolis. His father, Elwood, had dabbled in politics as a city alderman when Hubert Humphrey was mayor. A child of the Depression, Elwood Swanson was a simple man of extraordinary decency—honest, dependable, and, for a part-time politician, surprisingly nonpolitical. It was a legacy that Swanson's father received from *his* father, a Swedish immigrant who settled in Minnesota, built a profitable grocery business, raised six children, and served in the Minnesota state legislature.

As Swanson began to travel the world and meet with often skeptical Dow Corning executives who had little time to discuss ethics, he became intrigued by the possibility of linking the corporate bottom line with conscience and values. Realistically, could a corporation take its responsibilities to society and the environment as seriously as it took its sales and profits? Certainly there is an inherent conflict between a corporation's need to maximize profit and the desire to engage in socially responsible and ethical behavior. And Swanson knew of few organizations that had found an effective way to reconcile what could sometimes be two extremes. That was the intellectual puzzle that began to fascinate him. He started to view the assignment from Ludington as a challenge to subject the often abstract theories of ethics to a pragmatic test of corporate realities. How do you convert ethics from simple pieties on a piece of paper to a part of the ethos of a worldwide organization?

You start, thought Swanson, by recording the loftiest aims and goals of the people who worked at the company. In late 1976, he led the development of the company's first code of ethics, a brief document called "A Matter of Integrity," which was sent to every employee with a personal message from Ludington. It detailed the company's responsibilities to its employees as well as its employees' responsibilities to Dow Corning. It outlined proper relations with customers and suppliers, and it spelled out a number of ambitious conservation and environmental goals.

What would in time become, to Swanson, two of the most telling statements in the code were the declarations that (1) "Dow Corning will be responsible for the impact of its technology upon the environment...." And (2) We will continually strive to assure that our products and services are safe, efficacious and accurately represented in our literature, advertising and package identification. Product characteristics, including toxicity and potential hazards, will be made known to those who produce, package, transport, use and dispose of Dow Corning products."

For a company producing chemical products, these were

bold pronouncements. Still, what distinguished Dow Corning's ethics program from many others was its highly active and visible Business Conduct Committee, of which Swanson was the sole permanent member. The committee put teeth in the code, demonstrating to all employees that Ludington was serious about the effort. The system would eventually evolve so that up to six executives served three-year stints on the panel, devoting as much as 15 percent of their time to the job.

For a decade following its inception, the committee would conduct an average of about 25 audits annually. In the late 1980s and into the 1990s, the group would complete as many as 40 business audits a year around the world. In 1993, a new goal of reviewing every business operation every three years was put into place. These code of conduct reviews were face-to-face meetings with executives and managers that explored such sensitive topics as pricing issues, political contributions, bribes, payoffs, kickbacks, and conflicts of interest. They also were opportunities for the committee to keep the ethics issue alive and in the face of the company's leading managers.

Though the sessions occasionally uncovered serious misdeeds, they helped to make ethics a key component of Dow Corning's philosophy and culture. Swanson believed that for ethics to become credible, codes and values must be lived every day. The company had to reward ethically responsible behavior, deal firmly and visibly with ethics violations, and make ethics a regular part of the organization's communications. These small actions, consistently carried out, would ultimately forge an ethics-based culture. The face-to-face business conduct reviews, backed by ethics education programs and a semiannual employee opinion survey with an ethics section, served all those goals.

No less crucial, the meetings provided Swanson unusual exposure to all of the corporation's most talented managers and executives. At some point in their careers, they would either serve with him on the committee or sit on the other side of the table from him while a business audit was conducted. That made Swanson one of the few executives who knew

virtually every manager the company employed, a circumstance that often led Ludington to ask him to recommend
candidates for future business-conduct committee assignments.

What Swanson first assumed would be an assignment to
dish out management's flavor-of-the-month became a long-
term commitment. He saw Dow Corning's program as a noble
and informed effort, not window-dressing or an effort to gain
good will, not a program rushed into place to rehabilitate a
company with a tarnished reputation. With Ludington's strong
support, Swanson emerged as the initiative's leading propo-
nent and advocate. Through the years, he invested more and
more of his time in the ethics program. By 1990, he began to
devote nearly half his time to the program, making presentations on ethics to groups of employees, organizing audits, writing up audit reports for the committee and the board of directors, and updating the code to keep it vital and relevant. He
also managed, through his communications role, to assure
that ethical behavior and the company's code of conduct were
often referenced in speeches and presentations by Dow
Corning's senior executives. Through it all, he strove to build a
moral consensus inside the company that could guide employees to do the right thing.

In 1984, researchers from the Harvard Business School
were at the company's doorstep to gather information for what
would become a series of laudatory case studies on Dow
Corning's ethics program, now becoming a model for
Corporate America. Through speeches at business conferences and lectures at colleges, Swanson became a nationally
recognized expert on business ethics. "John Swanson was
much more genuine than most corporate ethics officers,"
thought Laura Nash, an ethicist at Boston University's
Institute for the Study of Economic Culture. "Many were limited in the way they looked at ethics. John had a comprehensive view that this was about a way of thinking. It seemed
much more tied to strategic issues than most. His program
had some teeth in it, too." Eventually, Swanson was asked to
be 1 of 13 members of the Arthur Andersen and Company

Advisory Council on Ethics, a group formed in 1987 to develop a comprehensive program to teach business school professors how to integrate ethics into mainstream business courses. Swanson was named co-chairman of the council in 1990.

Still, ethics was only part of Swanson's job. For most of his career, he directed Dow Corning's employee and management communications. He continued to write speeches for Ludington and other senior executives and to help them communicate internally with the company's more than 8000 employees.

In that capacity—long before he'd carved out his reputation in ethics—Swanson met an unusual Dow Corning chemist who, in the early 1970s, was abruptly transferred from the medical business into the communications department. His name was Silas A. Braley, and his sudden appearance in Swanson's domain became one of those small, random occurences that inadvertently ends up shaping every aspect of an individual's life. Someday, Swanson would regret ever meeting the man.

SPARE PARTS FOR THE BODY

Silas A. Braley had one of the world's most unusual job descriptions when he was dumped into John Swanson's communications department. The self-assured chemist was to tour the country as a corporate mouthpiece to promote the use of silicone body parts. Armed with a briefcase filled with artificial finger joints, ears, noses, chins, and breast implants, Braley would deliver a canned presentation dubbed "Spare Parts for the Body" to women's and civic groups, radio and television talk shows.

It was a bizarre assignment—and one that would have dramatic reverberations in the lives of John and Colleen Swanson—but the company would have been hard pressed to find a better spokesperson. A handsome man who dressed in dark suits, white shirts, and nondescript ties, Braley cut a convincing profile. A chemist by training, he was credible, even authoritative, about the medical applications for silicone. Like most of the chemists at Dow Corning, he was neither flashy nor flamboyant, so he hardly appeared as a promoter. "Si was thoughtful and quiet-spoken, an intellectual," says Eldon Frisch, a fellow Dow Corning chemist who had worked closely with Braley. "He was personable and worked hard to disseminate information about silicones."

If Braley easily impressed others with his knowledge of silicone, it was because he had already spent so much of his life involved with the chemical. Just after the war, he completed his studies in biology and chemistry at the University of Pittsburgh. While a student, Braley worked on a Dow Corning research project at the Mellon Institute, performing basic research on silicone rubber. He moved to Midland in 1950 to work as a chemist in Dow Corning's laboratories. His job: to help develop new products for the company's silicone rubber business. In 1959, after nine years in the same job, Braley moved out of the lab to help create Dow Corning's Center for Aid to Medical Research.

The center, with only a handful of staffers, was established to assist doctors who increasingly were contacting the company about using silicone for innovative and experimental medical applications. As executive secretary under a director, Braley rarely spent a day without being on the phone or meeting with an imaginative doctor wanting to get a few patents under his or her belt. Dow Corning wasn't in the business of designing new products. But it wanted to assist those who came to it with ideas, especially in the rapidly expanding medical arena.

One doctor reported placing an artificial urethra made of silicone rubber in a patient in the late 1950s. University of Michigan researchers made replacement bile ducts out of silicone. Typically, a doctor might read an article in an obscure journal about a silicone implant of one kind or another and then would call the company seeking advice on whether the substance could be used for other implants. "Essentially," says Braley, "what we said is, 'We don't know. We don't have any idea. Here's a sample. Try it in your animals and see what you think.'"

Braley served as the facilitator. He would work between the doctor and the chemists to come up with the right medical grade of material, effectively working both sides of the aisle, helping both the doctor and the company's objective to create new products and markets. Braley would routinely pass on general information on silicone, dispense advice on what physicians could and couldn't do with it, and hand out samples for research and experiments.

The center pursued dozens of uses for silicone. One doctor came to the company with the notion that burn victims might benefit from sitting in a bathtub filled with silicone fluid. He believed silicone would promote the healing of severe burns. Though the center helped the doctor with clinical research on the idea, the company found that victims treated with silicone still developed infections that often complicated treatment.

*   *   *

While plastic surgeons and doctors were getting more interested in using silicone, it was a substance little known to the general public. That is, until the media began writing about Carol Doda. A blonde topless dancer who did the Watusi at San Francisco's Condor Club in the mid-1960s, she helped to popularize the notion that, in her words, "A girl can be as large as her dreams." Doda attracted widespread media attention after a series of liquid silicone injections—not implants—transformed her from a rather ordinary go-go dancer with a 36-inch bust to a 44-inch topless superstar. "Science has invented all these new wonderful things," Doda told one reporter. "Why shouldn't we use them?"

Even though Dow Corning did not introduce its first breast implant until 1963, silicone may have found its way into the breasts of women as early as the late 1940s. In the aftermath of World War II, transformer coolant made of silicone was suddenly disappearing from the docks of Yokohama Harbor in Japan. The silicone fluid was used by cosmeticians to enlarge the small breasts of Asian prostitutes who knew that a more Western appearance would enhance their appeal to American servicemen. Larger doses of the doctored industrial fluids were injected directly into their breasts. To prevent silicone from migrating in the body, the Japanese added cottonseed or croton oil to cause immediate scarring, a way to contain the silicone at the site of injection.

Long before electronic gadgets and Toyotas, silicone injections became one of the first successful Japanese exports into America. The practice traveled immediately to Nevada, California, and Texas, where mostly exotic dancers sought out the procedure to increase the size of their breasts. Some doctors charged as much as $1000 to inject the fluid between the pectoral muscles of the chest wall and the back of the mammary tissues—a technique that became known as the "Sakurai formula" after a doctor who originated the practice in Japan. Dr. Sakurai moved to Beverly Hills, where he opened up a clinic and helped to popularize the injections in the United States. By 1965, the Food and Drug Administra-tion estimated that at least 75 doctors offered the treatment in Los Angeles alone. A doctor in Las Vegas crowed to *Newsweek* that he had given some 16,000 silicone injections to 200 women. Silicone "pumpers" trekked into Las Vegas to set up walk-in clinics in hotels along the strip. Complications due to injections soared so rapidly that in 1975 Nevada enacted emergency legislation making silicone injections a felony punishable by one to six years' imprisonment and a $10,000 fine. A year later, California passed a similar law making silicone breast injections a misdemeanor.

The uproar over silicone's dangers, however, failed to prevent continued use of silicone injections. An *Esquire* article in 1978 profiled an ex-con who traveled about the country injecting silicone into the breasts of thousands of women. He claimed to have injected more than 5000 over a 12-year period. "It's a lot like sculpting...." he said. "I form a picture in my mind of what someone's breasts could look like, really beautiful breasts I mean, and then I try to shape them to fit the image I have. That's a creative act, isn't it?" All told, perhaps as many as 50,000 American women and dozens of homosexual men—seeking to enlarge their penises—were injected with liquid silicone.

Predictably, horror stories abounded. Accidental injection of silicone into the bloodstream could result, albeit infrequently, in blindness and even death. Many women suffered gangrene, pneumonia, massive infection, and collapsed lungs. In some cases, silicone migrated to other parts of the body, accumulating in large lumps. Sometimes, the lumps could be surgically removed. In other cases, however, surgeons found them impossible to excise without undue disfigurement. At least four deaths were attributed to silicone abuse.

Sometimes, to avoid gangrene or the migration of infections to the brain and lung, surgeons had to perform mastectomies.

One 40-year-old woman who was treated by a self-styled "experienced silicone therapist" in the 1960s died hours after she was injected with a large syringe full of fluid under each breast. The silicone quickly traveled to her lungs and accumulated in such a heavy concentration that she ultimately suffocated. Another woman told *Ms.* magazine, the only woman's periodical that wrote skeptically of breast augmentation in its early days, that she was injected in the 1960s by a pediatrician at the age of 17. Unaware that silicone injections had never been approved for medical use, she signed the consent form that declared, among other things, "The procedure to be performed is experimental and unproved by medical experience." A year after she paid $50 a shot to have three ounces of silicone pumped into her breasts, she had to have a silicone lump in one breast aspirated and drained. Seven years later, both breasts had become painfully hard, and both nipples had collapsed.

Dow Corning claimed that it hadn't realized silicone was being used for breast injections until 1963, when Harvey D. Kagan, an osteopath who has been called the first real American apostle of breast enlargement through injection, spoke about his experiences at a convention of plastic surgeons. Kagan told the conference that he had been injecting women with a liquid silicone called Dow Corning 200 Fluid, a nonsterile industrial version, since 1946 on an experimental basis. He proclaimed his experiments "successful."

Alarmed by the news, Dow Corning began labeling the industrial fluid for manufacturing use only. The company also launched safeguards to prevent the injection of its sterilized, medical grade silicone, called Medical 360 Fluid, which was used as a lubricant for artificial joints and catheters. Dow Corning sold the fluid only to qualified physicians for what it called "valid research programs." Doctors who requested the fluid had to sign an affidavit stating that no silicones would be injected into human beings, as well as submit a statement describing their intended use of the fluid.

By 1964, the Food and Drug Administration got into the

act, declaring that the company's 360 silicone would be considered a "new drug" and could not be marketed without
undergoing testing. Still, it was virtually impossible for Dow
Corning to prevent some purchasers from falsifying the affi-
davits, or for that matter, buying industrial grade silicone in a
hardware store, attempting to sterilize it, and then injecting it
into women.

*   *   *

Ultimately, however, Dow Corning would be indicted by a
federal grand jury in 1967 for allegedly shipping an "unap-
proved drug" in interstate commerce in 1964 to Kagan and
other doctors. The company said it had no idea the doctors
planned to use the fluid for breast injections. Eventually, in
1971, Dow Corning pleaded no contest to the charges and
paid a $5000 fine. To offset the negative publicity, Braley was
called upon to hit the road with a Dow Corning public relations man to talk up the benefits of silicone with reporters and
editors around the country. "Si was an articulate, clever, and
witty individual," recalls Bob Emmons, who was then engaged
in public relations for the company's medical products. "Si
and I came up with a program to get the heat off of us. We
went to New York and called on the ladies' magazines with
press releases and other materials to get better publicity."

For his part, Braley was completely against silicone injections. "The doctors would be injecting it in large amounts," he
recalls, "and you would have globules of silicone fluid in there
even if it caused no reaction whatsoever, and we had no idea
whether it would or not. If it caused no reaction whatsoever,
you still would have a scar tissue forming around it, and you
still would have that scar tissue maturing and contracting, and
you would have a lumpy breast which would be impossible to
differentiate from a naturally occurring cancer."

A lawful alternative, however, was being thought up by a
young doctor sitting in a hospital laboratory in Houston,
Texas. In 1959, Frank J. Gerow was an enterprising resident

under Thomas D. Cronin, a surgeon at Baylor University.
Gerow was working late one night, waiting to fractionate
blood in the lab. In those days, residents and interns did virtually all of the lab work. The medical products industry had
only recently switched to storing blood in plastic bags rather
than the old sterilized bottles that hung from steady poles.
Sitting in the lab, with little to do except wait, Gerow began
kneading the plastic bag in his hand when it suddenly
occurred to him that it felt like a woman's breast. Why could-
n't they create a "falsie," he thought, a silicone bag filled with
some kind of fluid that could be implanted in a women's
breast?

Gerow knew all about the horrible history of liquid silicone
injections. He also knew that for decades bust-builders had
inserted an odd assortment of devices into women's breasts,
including small glass balls, plastic wool, ox cartilage, and various kinds of plastic sponges. None proved successful. The
implants either were not well tolerated or were reabsorbed by
the body, and some even caused cancer.

Both he and Cronin thought that if a saline solution could
be placed into a bag similar to the ones used to store blood, it
might make a good implant. Braley's Center for Aid to Medical
Research had just opened its doors in Midland, and a local
plastic surgeon who had studied with Dr. Cronin had gone to
the center's open house to hear Braley discuss the potential
for further medical uses of silicone. The surgeon, who practiced in nearby Saginaw, relayed word of the center to Cronin
in Texas and within weeks Braley heard from Cronin.

At Dow Corning, Braley fielded dozens of calls like this
from doctors all over the world who wanted to know if silicone
could be used for this or that. And Cronin's call was not the
first time a doctor had contacted him about using silicone for
a breast prosthesis. In the past, however, doctors had asked
about using the substance to create a sponge as a substitute
for normal breast tissue. Braley says he dissuaded them
because human tissue would inevitably grow into the sponge,
causing it to contract and disappear. The result, said Braley,
was that it eventually would become "a small hard lump."

The request from Cronin was different. The surgeon, who had a reputation as a cautious pioneer in plastic surgery, wondered if silicone could be used to create a bag that would hold a salt water solution. After writing a letter to Braley, Cronin dispatched his resident Gerow to Midland to discuss the use of silicone for the device. The Dow Corning chemists at the center were taken by him. Eldon Frisch, who also worked on the breast implant, remembers Gerow as "a dynamic person who pursued his ideas with a great deal of vigor." And at the very first meeting, ideas flew from him with ease and infectious enthusiasm. "We talked over many, many different things for plastic surgery," recalls Braley. "He was quite an inventive mind. And he was thinking about all kinds of different things, but the breast prosthesis was (the) main one we talked about at that time."

Gerow spent an entire week with Braley, exploring the possibilities of using silicone for chin and ear replacements, for cheek bones and other body parts. They chatted about the injection of silicone fluid to enlarge the breast. But it was the possibility of creating a breast implant that dominated most of the discussion.

Initially, Gerow had little interest in filling his bag with silicone. He preferred an inflatable silicone bag filled with the saline solution so that it could be adjusted to the size of the breast once placed into position by a surgeon. Braley disagreed. An inflatable implant made little sense, he believed, because it would be difficult to create a valve attached to the bag that wouldn't deteriorate over the years. Instead, he suggested the use of a silicone gel which would more likely, as he put it, "duplicate the feeling of the normal breast."

Though silicone gel had never before been used in a medical application, it was commonly accepted at Dow Corning that the gel was biologically inert. The company had been selling silicone fluids as a lubricant for hypodermic needles and as a skin lotion. Braley informed Cronin that a silicone gel would have the same chemistry as the bag and that he would expect "minimal reaction to it" by a woman's body. His belief in the safety of silicone was largely based on animal studies and on reports from doctors who used other silicone medical devices. A silicone brain-shunt had been used for years to drain fluid from the skulls of hydrocephalic children. A silicone band called the Scepters eye belt had been commonly placed around the eyeball for repair of retinal detachments. "The results coming back to us were so positive," says Braley. "We were getting no bad results at all. The doctors were uniformly positive about this. Silicone was the only soft material that had ever been accepted by the body."

Braley's assurances to Cronin and Gerow that silicone gel would be safe, however, were not based on clinical trials involving human beings. Nor were they based on animal studies using miniature implants. Cronin did perform some rudimentary dog studies of his own, putting miniature versions of the implants into no more than six dogs—two of which were studied for 18 months. But when autopsies were done on the animals, he did not do extensive microscopic studies of their organs. "At that time," Braley says, "there were no tests for implant materials. There was no protocol at the FDA. If you wanted to test a device for the FDA, how would you do it? Do you feed it to the patient? What do you do? You put it under the skin and look and see what happens. And that is what we had done in many, many cases—all of which reinforced the knowledge that these materials were satisfactory for use as far as we knew at that time and were infinitely superior to anything that was available as a substitute."

Over the next few years, the two doctors from Texas worked closely with Braley to create the first silicone breast implant. Braley worked up several versions of silicone bags and sent them down to Cronin, who implanted them in some animals. At a plastic surgeons' meeting in New Orleans, Braley brought the surgeon a jar filled with silicone gel so Cronin would have an idea of how it could work. "He stuck his finger in it and said, 'That looks and feels good,'" recalls Braley. Soon, Dow Corning was making several versions of the completed product and dispatching them to Texas. "Some were too hard or weren't the right shape," says Braley. "Or the edges on the molded bags were too sharp."

Finally, in early 1962, Braley supervised the making of the

first prototype in Dow Corning's fabrication laboratory. It resembled broad, slightly flattened cylinders molded together. They contained between a quarter and a third of a quart of milky-colored silicone gel. On the back of each prosthesis were small Dacron mesh patches that would adhere to the chest muscles to secure the implant without sutures. "They were very large, much larger than they are now," recalls Braley. "They had a thick wall and were quite hard compared to what we later made." Gerow installed the first pair of implants in a local woman in Houston in March of 1962, while Cronin and he were still performing their limited dog study.

The first operation was a success, and both doctors immediately began pressing Dow Corning for more implants. Braley helped convince Dow Corning's management that it should begin to sell silicone for medical applications. Before, the company had simply given it to selected doctors for free. The business of making the devices in volume was turned over to Dow Corning's new medical products division. "We crossed our fingers and hoped we wouldn't lose too much money," is the way Braley later put it.

Dow Corning launched its silicone breast implants in 1963 under the trade name Silastic®, making them available in eight sizes: mini, petite, small, small extra-fill, medium, medium extra-fill, large, and large extra-fill. No government approval was required, and the company had to meet no safety standards before putting the new medical device on the market. Though the Food and Drug Administration had overseen the regulation of pharmaceutical drugs since the early 1900s, it did not require premarket approval of medical products— even those placed inside the body. The FDA would not gain the authority to regulate medical devices until 1976, following the public furor over the Dalkon Shield.

So Dow Corning performed no safety tests of its own on the silicone breast implants, but instead relied on Cronin's limited, short-term studies. Indeed, three decades later, Braley would make a startling admission in a court deposition. Asked if he advised Dr. Cronin that the safety for the long-term use of silicone in human beings had not been established, Braley

said, "Sure...that's true. It had not been." After consulting
with Dow Corning's attorneys, however, Braley said the company had other test results and information that supported "the
probability that this material would be okay.... We certainly felt
that it was safe or we certainly would not have done it....[But]
there were no tests for implant materials either on the material or on the patient, on the animal. All we could do was put it
in and look and see what happens. There were no standards.
There were no protocols. There was nothing."

Cronin officially presented his paper on silicone breast
implants—detailing their creation and his belief that they
were safe—in late 1963 to the American Society of Plastic and
Reconstructive Surgeons, the professional group representing
the vast majority of board certified surgeons. The surgeon,
who had the appearance of a kind-hearted grandfather, delivered his findings in a slow Texas accent. He showed pictures
of the first woman ever implanted with silicone. His reputation as a conservative surgeon lent instant credibility to Dow
Corning's new product. Suddenly, a new business was born.
"After he gave his paper," recalls Braley, "we were inundated
with orders for implants and requests for silicone from plastic
surgeons." By 1967, one doctor at Johns Hopkins Hospital
estimated that more than 40,000 American women already
had silicone breast implants.

*   *   *

Si Braley's early and crucial involvement in the business
made him, in some odd way, its guardian and promoter. He
slowly emerged as Dow Corning's spokesperson for all silicone
medical applications. Unlike many of his anonymous colleagues in Midland, Braley was a well-known champion of silicone body parts. He cultivated strong ties to the rapidly growing numbers of plastic surgeons, not only in the United States
but also in such vanity capitals as San Paulo, Brazil. He met
with them in their offices, attended their conferences and
seminars, and always dazzled them with his expertise. "Si was

terrific," recalls Dr. James L. Baker, Jr., one of the country's most prominent plastic surgeons. "He was our guru. This guy knew more about silicone chemistry than probably anybody in the world. He really was a brilliant chemist. He worked with so many surgeons, and we formed close friendships. To us, Si *was* Dow Corning."

It wasn't only the plastic surgeons who grew to know and like him. Many journalists, particularly those writing the gee-whiz articles about silicone breasts that commonly appeared in many women's magazines, came to interview him for his thoughts on the subject. In a 1971 article in *Vogue* magazine, a writer dubbed him "silicone's guardian," and went on to say "a brilliant chemist who feels for silicone an almost anthropomorphic affection, Mr. Braley is affable and easy-going but adamant when it comes to keeping track of every pint of the fluid...."

Like many of the chemists at Dow Corning, Braley had an enormous ego. Many outsiders often referred to him as a doctor, though he had neither a Ph.D. nor an M.D. But he didn't go out of his way to correct the misimpression that led to much of his correspondence at the company being addressed to "Dr. Silas Braley."

By the time Braley was moved to Swanson's corporate communications staff in 1973, tens of thousands of women were having breast implants every year. Many implants were placed in women who had suffered breast cancer and had undergone mastectomies. Still, many more were placed in the breasts of women made self-conscious about their bodies by an increasingly vain society. Though some doctors worried about the cancer-producing potential of placing a foreign material into a part of the body that has shown a propensity to develop cancer, few had reason to question the safety of the breast implants or how long they might last. Gerow, who shared with Cronin the royalties on the device, would get up before the plastic surgeons at conferences and declare that some day archaeologists were going to dig up skeletons and find little more than two mounds of silicone and wonder what they were.

*   *   *

John Swanson knew that Braley was not happy with the transfer. For one thing, the Dow Corning veteran didn't believe he belonged in a communications department. He was, after all, a chemist who had been on the leading edge of an important technology breakthrough. He also felt Dow Corning was giving him a raw deal after all he had done to create a new market for silicones. But the center's business was winding down because silicone was no longer a new and rare substance. "The center had outgrown itself," says Frisch. "By then, the technology of silicones had become widely known. Computer-based searches of studies and research reports had become available, and Dow Corning had separate labs and facilities working on medical products."

In any case, an official job was created: Si Braley would be the public ambassador for the company's silicone applications for health care. When Braley left the center in 1973, only Frisch and a secretary remained. Though Braley may not have liked it, he had been playing the same role unofficially for years. The transfer, however, would lessen his contact with the surgeons and increase his exposure to the general public. He was a perfect choice for the job because he knew so much about silicone. He was the ideal pitchman for a confidence-building game, talking up the benefits of the company's full line of silicone body parts. At women's clubs, he tried to quell doubts that silicone posed significant health risks.

Swanson, of course, knew that Dow Corning had been in the breast implant business. But having Braley in the communications department made him far more knowledgeable about this small, and curious part of Dow Corning's business. It was certainly something of a novelty, and he mentioned it to Colleen, who was then his wife. She was an attractive 34-year-old brunette when he met her by chance at a Holiday Inn in her hometown of Petoskey, Michigan. Feisty and vivacious, Colleen was a compact woman, standing just 5-foot-1-inch tall and weighing just 105 pounds. She was there with a girl-friend and her parents, who were celebrating their wedding anniversary. Swanson was in town with Dow Corning colleagues on a weekend golfing trip that brought him to a course tucked into the northwest corner of the state.

Soon enough, the three-hour commute from Midland to Petoskey became a fixture in his life. He married Colleen in October of 1973, fewer than 4 months after they met. He had been divorced for 3 years, after a 10-year marriage that produced two children. Colleen, too, had divorced and had two children. Her first marriage had lasted 17 years, but many of those years were unhappy ones, and Colleen, was eager to put that life behind her and start fresh with John Swanson.

A month or so after marrying, the Swansons accompanied Braley and his wife, Mary Jane, to Detroit where Braley was to appear on Focus, a popular noon-time radio show on WJR hosted by J. P. McCarthy. The two couples drove the 125 miles from Midland to Detroit, after the show, had lunch together in the city, and then drove back and stopped in a nearby town for dinner. It was a long, full day, much of it filled with conversation about breast implants.

Colleen had long thought her breasts were too small—ever since her first pregnancy, when her breasts temporarily became much fuller and rounder. She felt self-conscious enough about it to wear a 32-B padded bra. When she flipped through clothing catalogs and scrutinized the female models in the advertisements, she would sometimes feel inadequate. More generally, Colleen had trouble finding clothes that would fit the upper part of her body—a reason why she often had to shop in teenagers' clothes departments.

But it wasn't until she prematurely gave birth to a son who died in 1963—just after President Kennedy's assassination—that she began to become more concerned about her appearance. She had carried her son for six months and a week when he was born weighing only three pounds. He lived two days. Her breasts were swollen and heavy with unneeded milk and wouldn't dry up. When they finally did, one was slightly larger than the other.

"My breasts were a mess," she says. "I felt very self-conscious about them. I was also a little bit insecure about it after

I married John. I had been through a traumatic divorce. My self-esteem was very low. I wanted to be as close to perfect as I could be."

Her interest in breast implants and her eventual decision to get them had nothing to do with childhood ridicule or the portrayal of feminine beauty on television or in women's magazines—all subtle forms of pressure that lead many women to plastic surgeons. It had nothing to do with general acceptance by others, even if the social psychology literature showed that cute infants were cuddled more often than homely ones, that attractive toddlers were punished less often, that the best-looking students got special attention from teachers, or that strangers typically offer help more readily to attractive people. And it had nothing to do with the Barbie doll, the plastic toy with dimensions that would translate to 40-18-32 if increased to life-size, even if feminists believe the doll has shaped teenage girls' attitudes about body image for generations. "I never had a Barbie doll when I grew up," says Colleen. "I was 16 before we had television. As I was growing up, no one ever made an issue of my breast size. I had more of a problem with glasses than my small breasts. I really didn't even think about the size of my breasts until after I had children."

She missed the fuller size of her breasts, and she wanted so badly to be perfect for her new husband. John Swanson thought his wife looked just fine. He was madly in love with her, and wasn't the least bit unhappy with the way she appeared. But after one failed marriage, Colleen Swanson was striving to make her second marriage perfect, to insure that her second chance at happiness would succeed where her first had not. So she listened intently to what Braley had to say, fascinated that something could safely be done to improve her appearance and allow her clothes to fit more comfortably.

Throughout that day with the Braleys, Colleen asked many questions, mostly related to the surgery itself: Could anything go wrong? How long was the recovery period? Was there a danger of the implants breaking? What would happen if something went wrong and they had to be replaced?

For nearly every question, thought Colleen, Braley had a

reassuring answer. "The implants, according to Si, were absolutely safe," she says, "no need to worry about anything. He told me silicone was totally inert and could not react with the human body in any way. It's difficult to recall with accuracy this many years after, but I can tell you that there were no negative answers."

Braley told her that most women who made the decision were housewives in their thirties—just like she—who gained both a psychological and physical uplift by having implants. Though Colleen didn't feel those were her main reasons for considering the operation, she thought these additional benefits sounded good.

Before their return to Midland, Braley said that if she decided to go ahead with the implants, he could personally recommend a plastic surgeon who was one of the very best in the country with the procedure. Braley, recalls Colleen, said he would be happy to talk with the surgeon to help arrange the operation.

Colleen thought long and hard about having the surgery, finally deciding in favor of it. Braley had given Swanson an actual implant so he could show it to her and she could see how it felt. She closely read the "Facts You Should Know About Your New Look" brochure that Dow Corning published. It was a relatively upbeat and positive brochure the company distributed to plastic surgeons, and it confirmed everything Braley said about the devices. The document posed commonly asked questions and provided answers that would reassure most women who might have had doubts about undergoing surgery for cosmetic reasons. Question: "How long will the mammary prosthesis last?" Answer: "Based upon laboratory findings together with human experience to date one would expect that the mammary prosthesis would last for a natural lifetime."

Swanson was himself convinced that if Colleen really wanted the implants, she should have nothing to fear. "Based on all I had learned it seemed to me there was nothing to worry about," says Colleen. "I had been advised by the one person who represented the best state-of-the-art knowledge of medical uses of silicone in the world. He knew the most competent plastic surgeons for this procedure in the United States. Dow Corning had originated the silicone implants and was a highly reputable organization. The long and short of it is that based on Si's reputation and Dow Corning's, I felt very confident that silicone implants were safe and that once implanted would last for the rest of my life."

Colleen Swanson decided to have the operation.

A SCULPTOR AND HIS CLAY

In late March of 1974, the Swansons packed Colleen's Chevrolet Impala convertible to the gills and headed south toward Florida on Highway 75 from their home in Midland. The trunk was loaded with suitcases filled with summer clothing: shorts and swimsuits for John, Colleen, and Colleen's two teenaged children. And one suitcase contained a small cardboard box with a pair of vacuum-sealed, sterile Dow Corning silicone breast implants. They were to be given to Dr. James L. Baker Jr. to replace the pair he was planning to stitch into Colleen.

This was a journey they would tell no one about, especially not the side trip to Dr. Baker. Not their closest friends, nor their own parents. This was, after all, a private matter. Colleen would have felt embarrassed if her parents or friends knew she was going to have a "boob job." Colleen would return to Midland, Michigan, with slightly larger breasts and nothing more. She would tell no one, and she would attract no extra attention to herself.

After a brief stop in Daytona Beach to visit his sister and parents, Swanson drove south to Orlando and Disney World. It would be a rather uneventful excursion, except for two incidents: Colleen's 16-year-old son, Kelly, got their car stuck in the sand on the beach as the tide rolled in, and Colleen went to Baker's office for her new look. Braley had paved the way for the trip shortly after Christmas by making a telephone call to the plastic surgeon. Baker followed up with correspondence to Braley and then with a February 4 call to

John Swanson, fixing a date of March 28 for the surgery, and agreeing to do the operation for only $100 if Swanson brought along the replacement pair of implants. Most surgeons were charging anywhere from $1000 to $3000 for the procedure.

A day before the surgery, Swanson checked into a motel near Baker's office on West Gore Street in Orlando. That afternoon, the Swansons went to meet the plastic surgeon for the first time. He had already sent Colleen prescriptions for antibiotics, vitamins, and blood work to speed up the process. So this initial visit was to allow Baker to go over the operation and put any remaining concerns Colleen might have out of her head. The moment she walked into the office of Drs. O'Malley, Douglas, Bartels, and Baker, she was impressed. Colleen was immediately greeted by a nurse who invited her into a well-appointed waiting room with soft, comfortable furniture. "You got the impression that he was successful, and the office was efficient," says Colleen.

Within minutes, Baker was escorting the Swansons into his office and talking about the details of the operation and the surgical options Colleen faced. Baker was a solidly built young man of 37 years with a warm, round face and blue eyes. He was almost arrogantly confident in his abilities as a surgeon, and perhaps he should have been, given Braley's enthusiastic recommendation.

Leaning back in a chair behind a desk, Baker took Colleen's personal history and heard what he often does from the patients who want breast implants: they want to look better. Like most of the women he had already operated on, Colleen was intelligent, attractive, neatly groomed. She wore a padded bra prior to surgery, and in clothes did not appear to have a noticeably small chest. In the interview, Colleen confirmed that she had enjoyed the enlargement of her breasts during her pregnancies and would like well-proportioned, "normal size" breasts. "She would like to be able to buy clothes that fit, and she is quite self-conscious of her small bustline," Baker later wrote in his pre-operative report.

He told Colleen that because of her short stature, he would probably use 200-cubic-centimeter implants, a size far below the then-maximum 340 cc models yet still considerably above the smallest 130 cc versions. If possible, however, Baker said he might go a little bit larger. The final decision could not be made until Colleen was on the operating room table and he had carved open the cavities into which the implants would be placed.

Baker informed the Swansons that he could use what he called the "infra mammary approach" in which he would install the implants through an incision in the crease of her breast. He had come to prefer this procedure to any other over the years because it was the easiest and most painless way to enlarge the breasts. Or, if Colleen preferred, he could install them through incisions in her armpits, a much more complicated operation. When these operations worked, Baker thought, they were great because patients had very little discomfort, they could go braless right after the surgery; and they had no scars on the breast. But it was difficult to make the breasts perfectly symmetrical, and the inch-and-one-half scars in each armpit often failed to heal properly.

Two other options, which Baker did not endorse, involved inserting the implants through the nipples or through two-inch circular cuts half way around the lower half of the areolas. These methods had the advantage of leaving a less conspicuous scar, but they also were slightly more complicated because they involved cutting through breast tissue—something Baker disliked doing because he didn't want to "violate" a part of the body with a high propensity for cancer. The Swansons decided in favor of the most common technique, inserting the implants through the bottom crease of the breasts.

After spending about 20 minutes going over such details, Baker quickly checked Colleen's breasts in an examination room to insure there was no evidence of existing tumors or cysts. Then, an assistant snapped preoperative photographs of her breasts. Before leaving the office, Colleen Swanson signed a carefully-worded consent form confirming that Baker had informed her of a list of potential difficulties:

a) That the operation has been done for several years, but the end results are not, and cannot be determined for a number of years to come.

b) That research indicates that the material does not cause malignancy in human subjects.

c) That there is a possibility that my body may not tolerate these implants, making it necessary to remove the implants, and that this occurs in a small percentage of cases.

d) That a cyst may form in the area adjacent to the implants, causing fluid accumulation which may require drainage by needle or removal of the implants.

e) That the breasts will feel firm for 3 to 6 months and possibly longer.

f) No guarantee has been given as to size and shape of the breasts. Good results are expected, but not guaranteed.

g) In some patients, the margin of the implants can be felt.

h) That there may be areas of anesthesia of the breasts and nipple erection may be impaired.

It read like any typical form a patient is required to sign before undergoing surgery or other medical procedure, the kind of form most people put their signature to after only the most cursory reading. Reassured by Baker of the operation's success rate, Colleen had no doubts at all about going through with it. "He told me the procedure was relatively safe," she recalls. "I only had two things to worry about: infection or if I were in a car accident and the implant ruptured. I know I thought he was confident, or I never would have let him touch me."

Her surgical appointment was set for exactly 8 A.M. the next day.

*   *   *

Though recommended by Braley, Baker had not yet established his reputation as one of the country's leading plastic surgeons. By the mid-1980s, *Harper's Bazaar* would award him an "honorable mention" as one of the nation's outstanding surgeons in the field of breast augmentation. By 1995, after putting breast implants in more than 4000 women, including his own teenaged daughter, he would be named president of the American Society for Aesthetic Plastic Surgery.

Baker, now silver-haired and more rotund, is witty and out-going. He speaks as matter-of-factly about surgery as a minister might speak about the Bible, routinely communicating the most intricate details of cutting into tissue or whacking off bone that would make many cringe. He wears a sparkling white smock over a striped white shirt and gray slacks. His name is stitched in bright red lettering over his left breast. He speaks on the subject of plastic surgery with authority and he speaks fast, like a machine gun spewing words instead of bullets.

"Cosmetic surgery," believes Baker, "is a very selfish proce-dure. People do it because they want to look better. Many women who get implants felt they never looked good in their clothes. They always felt unfeminine. They started comparing breast sizes when they were children, just as men compare penis sizes. Most women who want breast implants simply want to look normal. The comment I always get is, 'I don't want to look like Dolly Parton'. Yet if there was an operation to make a man's penis bigger, I could guarantee you that every man who came in would want the El Grande Supremo model. But the women don't want to be big, big."

Twenty years earlier, however, he was a relative newcomer to a still new field of surgery. Baker had received his board certification from the American Board of Plastic Surgery in 1973, only a year before Colleen came to him for implants. Yet, even then, what he lacked in experience he more than made up for with ambitious enthusiasm. An enterprising sur-geon, Baker quickly impressed colleagues with his dedication to knowing more about breast implants and why women get them. The information inserts Dow Corning packaged with its implants referenced his clinical studies on the devices. The company even funded his first educational film on the proce-dure. It was made in 1972 with a $500 grant, and would even be shown on the *Phil Donahue Show* in the late 1970s to pro-mote breast implants over liquid silicone injections.

A decade after Dow Corning entered the business, breast implants were fast becoming one of the most frequently requested cosmetic operations in the United States. Women's magazines such as *Vogue* and *Harper's Bazaar* carried stories with such titles as "The Perfect Bosom" or "Breast Sculpture" written in superlatives by writers who saw few downsides to the operations. Some of these articles elevated plastic surgeons to near hero status. "If plastic surgeons are the sculptors of the medical world, then the female breast is very special clay, capable of being transformed into a more beautiful expression of itself," wrote one journalist in *Harper's Bazaar.*

Baker was fast building a reputation as an expert sculptor and researcher. Just five months before the Swansons arrived in his office, he stood before the American Society of Plastic and Reconstructive Surgeons in Hollywood, Florida, to deliver a paper on the "psychosexual dynamics" of women who received breast implants. The rising demand for the procedure, Baker said, indicated that "there are thousands of women with feelings of inadequacy about the size of their breasts....The size and shape of the woman's breasts are extremely important to her body image and her concept of self."

Baker's study—based on interviews with 10 of his own patients as well as 132 women who had undergone the operation with one of the other three doctors in the Orlando practice—would later become one of several studies used by plastic surgeons in an effort to redefine small breasts as a medical disease requiring treatment. Baker, for example, found that

> adolescence was marked by feelings of inadequate sexual development, when the patient became aware of the differences between her breast development and that of her peers. Self-consciousness about her breasts inhibited breast play. Many reported never undressing in front of men, and having intercourse only in the dark. Disturbances in marital relationships were common. Two patients reported they could not experience orgasm. Three of the five married

women reported marital infidelity, seeking affirmation of their attractiveness to men.

Backed by such studies, in 1982 the American Society for Plastic and Reconstructive Surgery filed formal comments with the Food and Drug Administration that, incredibly, called small breasts "deformities." Though the statement was later repudiated by the plastic surgeons, it was a bold attempt to vastly expand the market potential for breast implants by getting cosmetic surgery fully covered by medical insurance. The plastic surgeons' group argued that: "There is a substantial and enlarging body of medical opinion to the effect that these deformities are really a disease which in most patients results in feelings of inadequacy, lack of self-confidence, distortion of body image, and a total lack of well-being due to a lack of self-perceived femininity. The enlargement of the under-developed female breast is, therefore, often very necessary to insure an improved quality of life for the patient."

Much to his amusement, Baker also discovered something else in his "psychosexual" study of 1973. He found that women who undergo a breast implant operation often minimize the risks even when they are thoroughly described by plastic surgeons, who relied on Dow Corning and other makers to inform them of the downsides. It was a finding, believes Baker, that has much relevance today to charges by many patients that they were never fully informed of the potential dangers of silicone. "They hear what they want to hear," insists Baker. "The patients were often in denial." Baker says that after he listed a series of risks involved with the operation, the patients in his study were sent to a psychiatrist who asked the women if they could remember what they were told could go wrong. "Most of them answered no," recalls Baker. "Some suggested I told them it might cause cancer. But I told them it would not cause cancer. So they had that backwards, and the rest of it they totally misunderstood. They repressed the negatives about breast implants because they only wanted to hear the positives."

*   *   *

Baker's interest in the plastic surgery field surfaced early in his life. As a youngster, Baker found himself fascinated by Walt Disney's animated movies—so much so that he desperateley wanted one day to work in Disney's studios as a cartoonist. But at the age of 11, he was riding his bicycle down a steep hill in Somerville, New Jersey, when suddenly the front wheel fell off. Baker tumbled over the handlebars and landed on his face. The country doctor who treated him suggested that his parents might want to take the child to a plastic surgeon in New York to repair the probable scarring on his face, but the Bakers didn't have the money for such a luxury. "I had a lot of scars and was in therapy for three or four years," says Baker, who still bears a small, one-inch scar from the accident below his left nostril.

The accident, however, proved something of an epiphany. "I then thought, 'I love medicine and I love to work with my hands.' Plastic combined art and surgery together. So that satisfied me. From the time I was 11, I wanted to be a plastic surgeon." After spending a year at the University of Miami's Medical School, he transferred to the University of Amsterdam in The Netherlands where he earned his M.D. in early 1964. He returned to the United States for a four-year residency in general surgery at Monmouth Medical Center in New Jersey. From 1965 to 1969, he spent most of his hours in operating rooms assisting and doing all kinds of surgeries from tonsillectomies to cyst removals. It was during the latter part of his final two-year residency in plastic surgery at Orange Memorial Hospital in Orlando, however, that he witnessed what was for him a turning point.

At a cosmetic surgery symposium in Miami, in February 1971, Baker intently watched Dr. John Williams, a plastic surgeon based in Beverly Hills, perform a breast augmentation as an outpatient procedure on a woman under local anesthesia. At the time, it was highly unusual, Baker had been trained to do implant surgery under general anesthesia in a hospital. "We then tied the patients down in beds for five days," he says.

"They weren't allowed to move their arms. They had to be fed by the nurse. They weren't allowed to get out of bed. We bound them all and they were laying down with their arm restraints on so they couldn't lift a finger. You didn't want them to move their muscles under their arms to prevent bleeding."

But Dr. Williams dispensed with all the cautionary procedures, cut open and stitched his patient under local anesthesia, and sent her on her way. "The patient got off the operating table, they walked her out, put her in a wheelchair, and she went home," remembers Baker. "They brought the patient back the next day, and she walked in on her own and seemed happy and was moving her arms. She had a tight sweater on and she looked great. I thought I had seen a miracle, honest to God."

Baker rushed back to Orlando and eagerly told the highly conservative chiefs of surgery at Orange Memorial what he had seen, suggesting that they begin doing breast implants on an outpatient basis. "They looked at me with those jaundiced eyes because I was always coming in to them with new ideas, and they just shook their heads at me," says Baker. "They said, 'Why don't you work it out and after you do 20 of them let us know' and kinda laughed. They thought that was really crazy."

Undeterred, Baker asked the nurses in the hospital's nursing pool if they knew women who wanted free breast implants—so he could perfect the outpatient technique. "I got a lot of takers and started doing them in the hospital," he recalls. "They seemed to be doing great. They didn't have as much pain as the other patients who were tied down. They looked a lot better, and we found you didn't need the dacron patches to stick [the implants] to the chest wall."

Soon after completing his residency, Baker joined the private practice of his surgery chiefs and convinced them to convert a large janitor's closet into a small operating room so he could perform outpatient breast implants at $1000 a pair. In 1971, Baker became the first plastic surgeon in Florida to do cosmetic surgery in an office. Before long, says Baker, "we just got a ton of them." Patients liked the idea of avoiding a hospital stay because it would make it less likely for friends and others to know they were having their breasts done. The procedure could be performed more cheaply since hospitalization was not required. And the recuperation period was not nearly so long.

No less critical, the cramped quarters of the former janitor's closet left little room for more than the patient, a surgeon, and a nurse. The room was so small that Baker couldn't fit a stretcher in it along with the operating table. So Baker, who also was without his own resident, learned to perfect the breast enlargement operation largely unassisted. He would start the IV for sedation, quickly inject the patient with a local anesthetic, mark her, and then run out to wash his hands. When he returned, his nurse would help him gown and glove, after which he would drape the patient and do the operation himself. The nurse stood there, chatting to the woman on the table, ready to administer a bit more anesthetic if needed. "So I learned to do augments without any assistance at all," says Baker.

Bolstered by his success, the industrious surgeon sought funding from Dow Corning to make the educational film that could be shown to other surgeons to popularize the procedure. In the film, Baker, swathed in surgeon's whites, can be seen installing a pair of implants in a 21-year-old woman with blonde hair. He did the operation just as he had seen it done two years earlier: under a local anesthetic on an outpatient basis. Baker still recalls "this little girl, waving good-bye to us, driving away in a Volkswagen. She was my movie girl." A story that long made the rounds of Dow Corning has it that when the 16mm film was later shown to the board, one of the directors abruptly left the boardroom sick to his stomach.

When Baker opened his own private practice in 1977 in posh Winter Park, Florida, a nationwide boom in plastic surgery was underway. Upward of a million Americans were getting themselves snipped, sculpted, tucked, and reshaped every year. Some observers believed the "plastic explosion," as *Time* magazine called it, was being spurred by the self-improvement obsession of the 1970s. In truth, new technology made it easier to do even more cosmetic surgery at more affordable prices in a doctor's office, instead of a hospital or medical center. A widespread, unbridled belief in the promise of science and technology collided with an increasingly self-conscious and vain society.

Cosmetic surgery was coming out of the closet. Vast numbers of Americans were willing to go under the knife for the sake of vanity, some as easily as if going to a hair stylist for a new cut. Once a secret indulgence of rich dowagers and aging actors, face lifts were fast becoming a middle-class status symbol. Clerks, salespeople, and secretaries were using vacation days and credit cards to have tummies tucked, droopy eyelids tightened, and immense noses whittled down to size.

Of all the enhancing tricks in a surgeon's tool kit, breast enlargement was one of the fastest growing. After all, the contour of the female breast has been glorified in paintings and sculpture for centuries. To many men and women in Western society, breasts were the most visible characteristic of a woman, the very symbol of femininity. Finally, plastic surgeons with silicone-filled bags offered hope for the flat-chested.

Breast augmentation was also, of course, a new and welcome source of additional income for the surgeons. It was a fast and relatively easy operation to perform—and it was highly profitable. A competent surgeon could do as many as half a dozen of the procedures in a single day, if he could find enough women willing to undergo the operation.

Baker's timing in opening his own practice seemed perfect. He invested $800,000 to build his own surgical suite in the basement of a new building on West Morse Boulevard, just a stroll away from Winter Park's elite shopping district. His new operating room was at least three times the size of his old janitor's digs cum-surgical suite. There was a recovery room, as well as three generously sized patient bedrooms with TVs for overnight stays. In those early days, when he was in his forties and building his practice, Baker's operating room had the efficiency of a modern factory. In a single day, he would sometimes perform five or six implants, a face lift, a nose job, and eyelid surgery, wielding a scalpel from the morning until 10 at night.

He worked incredibly long hours, quickly establishing himself in the field by contributing myriad articles to the leading journals on plastic surgery, becoming a frequent speaker at annual conferences of plastic surgeons, and serving on numerous committees of the two largest professional organizations for plastic surgery. In the process, he created a widely used classification scale to allow surgeons to judge the hardness of breast implants, which sometimes have to be removed because of capsular contracture—the formation of a capsule of scar tissue around the implant.

He also became credited with inventing a nonsurgical procedure to break up such scar tissue. The procedure was the result of an unusual experience with a patient in 1975. At the time, Baker had scheduled a surgery to replace the implants of a patient whose breasts had become unbearably hard. Two days before her scheduled surgery, however, she had gone to a party where she met a professional football player who had known her during her university days. "He sees her, runs up to her and grabs her and does a bear hug, and they hear this pop," says Baker. "Of course, these two big torpedoes were sticking in his biceps. He said, 'What was that?' She said, I think my beads broke, and ran into the bathroom and her breasts were soft." The upshot: Baker found that physically manipulating the breasts might rupture the scar membrane, loosen the tightness of the implant, and eliminate the need for surgery. The breast is grasped tightly in both of the surgeon's hands. Maximum pressure is exerted and the hands are rotated 360 degrees, so that the expanding implant inside the women's breast literally ruptures the fibrous capsule in all directions. Years later, Dow Corning would advise surgeons against the practice, for fear that it would rupture the implant as well, spilling silicone gel out of it and into the body.

*   *   *

On March 28, 1974, five months after marrying John Swanson, Colleen lay flat on her back on a black-topped table under a bright lamp in Baker's cramped operating quarters. It was just after 8 A.M. Baker, assisted by a nurse, had already marked a center point in the creases of her breasts exactly six centimeters below her nipples. He generously painted her breasts and chest walls with Betadine, the copper-colored antiseptic. Baker sedated Colleen intravenously with Valium and then injected the incision areas in the creases of both her breasts using Xylocaine with Epinephrine, a potent anesthetic. After still another prepping with Betadine, the patient was draped and finally ready for the operation.

Baker quickly left the room to wash his hands again in a sterile solution and just as quickly returned. He picked up his scalpel and cut under one breast, then the other, roughly two centimeters on each side of the point he had drawn earlier. After slicing through the skin and subcutaneous tissue with the scalpel, he inserted a rake-like surgeon's tool into the open wound to lift each breast from the chest wall. Baker meticulously cauterized the exposed blood vessels with electric current to prevent them from bleeding after the operation, a circumstance that could cause dangerous swelling.

Then, with confident precision, he created a cavity for each implant by bluntly inserting his gloved fingers through the incisions. The cavity needs to be of generous size, for if the implants are forced into a tight fit, they are likely to be much too firm, pressured by the surrounding tissues. Baker cleaned out each cavity with a saline solution as his assistant opened up Dow Corning's film-wrapped sterile package to remove a pair of 235-cubic-centimeter implants. Baker then lifted each breast with a stainless steel retractor and pushed the folded implant through the small incision, using only his fingers, to prevent any tear in the implant's envelope. Within minutes, he completed his sutures, closing each wound in three layers and applying only small bandages over the closed incisions. Colleen was soon on her way home in a support bra.

All told, the operation took no more than 45 minutes. In his operative report, Baker wrote that "patient tolerated the procedure well and was discharged in good post-operative condition." Colleen, however, was surprised by how badly she started to hurt as soon as the anesthetic began to wear off. Walking back to her motel room from the parking lot, she felt so much pain in her chest that she had to stop to sit on a step. She began crying, prompting one concerned guest to ask if she needed any help. When the Swansons finally reached their poolside room, Colleen went directly to bed. The next day, Swanson took the children to Disney World while Colleen stayed behind in the motel.

For the next three days, Colleen confined herself to the room. Although the pain from the operation was numbed by medication prescribed by Dr. Baker, she also felt constant nausea. Her breasts were obviously larger. Maybe, she thought, they were a little too large. But it was hard to tell so soon after the procedure. On April 1, four days after the operation, the Swansons returned to Baker's Orlando office for a final checkup before departing for home. Baker apparently was pleased with his handiwork. "Patient has had beautiful results," he wrote in his clinical records. "Steristrips reapplied to the incision areas. No evidence of hematoma, seroma, infection. Final instructions given. The patient returning to Michigan. To remove steristrips in two weeks at home."

John and Colleen Swanson and her two teenagers drove home, straight north up Highway 75, with an evening stay in a roadside motel. But Colleen was still experiencing chest pain and nausea when the car reached the driveway of their home on Fuller Drive in Midland. She was a 32-C, a full cup size larger, but she was also weary and exhausted from it all. "I can remember when we arrived home that night my neighbor was outside, and she said, 'Oh you look awful.' I said 'it was a long, tiring drive.'"

Swanson helped her inside, and she stayed there for days, never leaving the house.

THE MARKET GROWS AND THE QUESTIONS BEGIN

There is at least one axiom in business that has always stood the test of time and always will. Success breeds competition, even in a niche business as unique as silicone breast implants. At just about the same time that Silas Braley began touring the country to talk up the benefits of silicone body parts and Colleen Swanson made her own decision to get new breasts, Dow Corning found its breast implant business under attack by smaller and more aggressive entrepreneurs.

Heyer-Schulte, a tiny medical devices company in Goleta, California, lured five young scientists and salesmen from Dow Corning in 1972 to launch itself into the breast implant business. The group, led by former Dow Corning chemist Donald K. McGhan, used their experience to help Heyer-Schulte develop cheaper and softer versions of implants to compete directly with Dow Corning. Two years later, in 1974, McGhan left Heyer-Schulte to start his own company, McGhan Medical Corporation in Santa Barbara, California. McGhan's notion was to build upon the basic technology developed by Dow Corning to make implants that more closely resembled the human breast by putting more liquid silicone gels into thinner envelopes or shells.

Dow Corning's original products looked like breasts when they were placed on a table. They were heavy silicone bags that contained thick, cohesive gel. "The problem was that when the patient lay down, her breasts looked like Mount

Vesuvius," recalls Dr. James Baker. "Some female plastic surgeons were saying, 'Look guys, you may know what a female
breast looks like vertical. But you sure don't know what one
looks like horizontal because it becomes a pancake.'" Dow
Corning's competitors, Heyer-Schulte and McGhan, listened
to the complaints and learned from them how to develop
implants that looked and felt more real than Dow Corning's
products.

Suddenly, Dow Corning not only found its business under
assault from two pesky California entrepreneurs, but it also
found itself losing significant business to these companies as
plastic surgeons began to prefer the new, more natural look of
the products being sold by Heyer-Schulte and McGhan
Medical. By 1975, Dow Corning estimated that it once
monopolistic market share had fallen to about 35 percent as
still more plastic surgeons dropped its product in favor of the
competition. In some cases, Dow Corning's new rivals slashed
prices—to as low as $100 a pair, when Dow Corning was
charging $220 a pair—to win over some of the most promi-
nent surgeons, including Dr. James Baker.

Alarmed by the dramatic loss of market share, Dow
Corning hurriedly assembled a task force in early 1975 to create a new generation of implants. Art E. Rathjen, a large bull-
dog-like man with a brusque voice and a natural frown, was
selected to lead the task force. He was hard-driving and domi-
neering, and his Dow Corning superiors knew that if anyone
could get the new product to market on schedule it was
Rathjen. He boasted to one friend that during his stint in the
military he would walk the grounds of a boot camp with a
swagger stick, rapping new recruits on their heads. To
acquaintances and colleagues who didn't know him well, he
appeared intimidating. His friends, however, could attest that
under all his bluster, Rathjen had a warm and sensitive side.
In any case, in this assignment he would set strict deadlines,
cajole people to move faster, and, in the records of the task
force meetings, would count down the weeks, days, hours, and
even minutes to the launch date of the new products.

Rathjen would later become the only non-doctor to hold

membership in the American Society of Plastic and Reconstructive Surgeons by serving as the group's official photographer. It was rumored at one time that his photography budget at Dow Corning exceeded the travel budgets of some of the company's sales reps. Initially, Rathjen traveled to myriad conferences and seminars to snap candid photos of plastic surgeons at the meetings with a Nikon camera. He then would send a pair of eight-by-ten glossies to each photographed doctor, asking the surgeon to autograph one of the pictures and return it to him in Midland. In a brief note, Rathjen would write that he had long been a fan of the physician's work. It was ass-kissing salesmanship at its finest. Over the years, he also clicked hundreds of pictures of women before and after their implant operations. Indeed, in one court battle, Dow Corning's lawyers would complain that the opposition attempted to characterize Rathjen as a "pervert" by grilling him about his numerous photographs of patients' breasts.

Rathjen gathered his task force for the first time on January 22, 1975, in "the orange room"—so named because of the color of the walls—on the second floor of Dow Corning's former corporate headquarters on South Saginaw Avenue. The group included five company insiders and four active consultants. True to form, Rathjen immediately set an exceptionally short deadline for the new product: June 1, little more than four months away. The goal: To develop a new series of implants with varying "profiles" filled with "flo-gel," or more watery silicone gel, in a new sterile package.

The task force agreed to meet weekly, every Friday morning from 8 to 10 A.M. Assignments were handed out to meet rigid timetables for production changes, the creation of the new envelopes and gel, packaging, and marketing plans, as well as some minor testing of the new product.

Rathjen and Dow Corning did not believe extensive medical testing was necessary because the new implants would still be based on materials substantially similar to those used in the company's first generation of implants developed by Braley, Gerow, and Cronin. But one potentially troublesome question that immediately arose was whether a new softer gel would leak, or bleed through the thinner envelope at a greater rate than the current models. Two chemical engineers, William D. Larson and Thomas D. Talcott, were asked to explore this issue, among others.

Within four days of the first meeting, Rathjen noted that the task force had only two weeks before the new gel was to be formulated and the filling of envelopes was to begin. "A question not yet answered is whether or not there is an excessive bleed of the gel through the envelope," Rathjen wrote in a memo to his colleagues. "We must address ourselves to this question immediately, determine what the facts are, and decide whether the plant is to proceed with the filling of the current inventory. Question: Does the new proposed mammary bleed any more than our standard product? If the product does bleed more, is it substantial enough that it will affect the product acceptance? A 'go or no go' decision will have to come from the Business Board. The stakes are too high if a wrong decision is made."

The same question would seem to come up again and again. It arose at the group's next meeting on January 31, when both Talcott and Larson informed Rathjen that the data on gel bleed were not yet complete. Five days later, however, the pair sent a memo to the task force: "We are concerned about a possible bleed situation as we are about the safety test results, about the suitability of the new gel in the contour-shaped prosthesis and simultaneously introducing a complete new line of sterile products," they wrote. Yet, the two chemists unofficially concurred that they thought the new gel would bleed no more than the gel Dow Corning had been using since the early 1960s. So the company eventually decided to go ahead with it. In his minutes of the meeting, Rathjen began to note the countdown to his deadline: "17 weeks, 121 days, 2,904 hours, and 174,240 minutes."

As marketing drew up its plans and the chemists performed tests to determine whether the new implants leaked more silicone than previous models, animal testing of the new devices was begun by an independent laboratory. A seven-day test by Biometrics found "mild to occasionally moderate acute inflammatory reaction" in animals but the lab believed it was not possible to tell whether it was due to the trauma of inserting the implant or the silicone itself. Tests on three monkeys implanted with the new devices found "some migration" of the new gel in their bodies, but no real concern seemed to surface about that finding. After all, Rathjen and virtually everyone else involved in the project believed that silicone was biologically inert. If it bled from the envelope in small quantities and migrated to other parts of the body, they believed, it still was not going to cause any harm. Even so, at the group's February 7 session, the marketing manager, Tom Salisbury, recommended that the company bring out its new implants with its current gel until field clinical evaluations could be completed because of the "questionable appearance" of the new implant with the new gel. The recommendation was accepted by the task force.

Throughout the process, Rathjen cracked the whip constantly. "He was a bulldozer," recalls Talcott. "There was a lot of pressure on us to get the new product out." He left nothing to chance, issuing tough memos that barked orders demanding that every deadline be met. Wrote Rathjen in the group's February 14 minutes: They "have got to decide *now, right now,* what is or is not a satisfactory envelope." Another chemical engineer who served as secretary to the group, Ann Berg, added to the pressure to speed development of the new implants. "With the changes in the plastic surgery business that are happening, RIGHT NOW (McGhan Medical, Heyer-Schulte, etc.) it was felt that aggressive development and marketing activity in the next four months will make a tremendous difference in Dow Corning's position in this market," wrote Berg. "The time to act is NOW."

By mid-May the task force was making amazing progress allowing the marketing staff to show the new implants at a California plastic surgeons' meeting on April 21, six weeks ahead of schedule. The company had already produced 10,000 pounds of the new gel. But already competitors, such as McGhan, were saying that Dow Corning's new product "was not of good enough quality to pass their quality control" standards. Salisbury, the

Dow Corning marketing rep on the task force, was concerned that the new implants appeared "oily" after being manipulated. He even suggested that salesmen frequently clean demonstration samples with soap and water in washrooms before showing them to surgeons.

Still, by May 23, Dow Corning had received orders for 500 pairs of the new implants, 200 of which were from competitive accounts, even though Berg expressed some doubts over whether the quality of the product was improved enough for it to be sold.

As the manufacturing plant geared up for the launch of the new implants in September 1975, it was running extraordinary rejection rates for quality. "Reject rate has been high," according to one internal memo. "Some lots have suffered a 50 percent reject rate at inspection. One lot of 1000 units was totally rejected. Reasons for reject have been floating dirt; weak bags, and embedded dirt." Even though the new implants hadn't officially been introduced, at least 11 of them already had been returned by doctors because of quality problems by September 22.

At a breast symposium for plastic surgeons in October 1975 in Scottsdale, Arizona, two of the company's new implants embarrassingly ruptured during augmentation surgery for a video-taped demonstration. Talcott was nearly beside himself. "When will we learn at Dow Corning that making a product 'just good enough' almost always leads to products that are 'not quite good enough'?" wrote Talcott in a memo to Rathjen. "During our task force assignment to get the new products to market, a large number of people spent a lot of time discussing envelope quality. We ended up saying the envelopes were 'good enough' while looking at gross thin spots and flaws in the form of significant bubbles. The allowable flaws are written into our current specifications."

Soon, several salesmen in the field were sending letters back to headquarters grousing about the quality of the new implants. In March of 1978, Frank Lewis, Dow Corning's sales rep in Detroit, complained to the home office about "an excessive number of ruptures" over the past six months. He told of a telephone call from a plastic surgeon at Henry Ford Hospital in Detroit who experienced four consecutive ruptures of Dow Corning products as he tried to put them into the breasts of a patient. Ultimately, the doctor used a Heyer-Schulte implant instead. For Lewis, it was not an isolated problem. At least two other doctors who were clients were evaluating competitive products because they noticed a difference in the new envelope Dow Corning was using. Some of Lewis's surgeons experienced rupture rates ranging from 11 percent to 32 percent with the new implants. "Now we face losing the business at Henry Ford due to ruptures," wrote Lewis. "I find it difficult to comprehend that I am the only one experiencing a rupture problem of this proportion. All of the above doctors have made the same comment: 'Noticing a difference in our envelope.'...I have lost more business recently due to ruptures than I lost last year due to competitors' sales efforts."

Similar memos came into the company from other locations. Cran Caterer, a sales rep in Chicago, complained that a doctor who typically used 70 pairs of implants a year experienced two consecutive ruptures in the middle of an operation. "The doctor said he implanted the first side with no problems and as he was handling (the) prosthesis to put in (the) other side it ruptured in his hand," wrote Caterer in a January 21, 1977, memo. The backup implant, meantime, was leaking gel out the side. The doctor was so concerned that he removed the implant already installed in the patient and used a pair of implants from a competitor.

Wooing back plastic surgeons who had already switched to competing products sometimes proved difficult—especially because of the belief by many surgeons that Dow Corning's use of thinner envelopes and more liquid gel contributed to rupture problems. In one instance, a Dow Corning sales representative trying to win back Dr. Fred Grazer of Newport Beach had given him three pairs of new implants for evaluation. Grazer, a prominent plastic surgeon who was doing 400 implants a year, had switched to a Dow Corning competitor after having problems with the company's quality. But all six of the new gel-saline implants, according to an internal memo, were "greasy" with "excessive gel bleed." Grazer was so upset the sales rep called him "downright indignant." "The thing that is really galling is that I feel like I have been beaten by my own company instead of the competition," wrote Bob Schnabel, the salesman to his Dow Corning boss. "To put a questionable lot of mammaries on the market is inexcusable. I don't know who is responsible for this decision but it has to rank right up there with the Pinto gas tank." Schnabel was referring to the controversy over the safety of Ford Motor Company's Pinto car. Critics alleged that the location of the car's fuel tank in the rear of the car made the Pinto a firetrap. Dow Corning would later say that a review of its records showed that Schnabel's complaint was the only one involving this lot of implants. "The salesman's language over-dramatizes an isolated incident," according to the company.

But there were many complaints. Within months of the product launch, plastic surgeons around the country began to express concerns that the new envelopes seemed to bleed more gel than the earlier models. Frank Gerow, who with Cronin invented the silicone implant, called to relay the fears of some surgeons at the Scottsdale meeting that "something is coming through the envelope to the tissue." Gerow told Talcott that patients experienced less contracture or hardening of the breasts with the older, firmer gels. "He concludes we need a 100 percent tied up gel now, and encouraged work on such a gel," wrote Talcott to his colleagues. "I'm inclined to agree that something may be coming from the envelope, but I'd question—could it be miscellaneous contamination during our manufacturing process?"

Talcott never did get an answer, or at least an answer that satisfied his concerns. Ultimately, he quit the company in protest in 1976 after 24 years with Dow Corning. Talcott claimed the new breast implants the company was selling could rupture and leak, posing a serious health risk. He worked for two other implant makers after leaving Dow Corning, and then started his own materials consulting business in 1982. Dan Hayes, CEO of Dow Corning Wright, would later say that Talcott "left as a disgruntled employee. You've got to question to some degree his motive (for speaking out against the company)."

Nonetheless, Rathjen himself was now voicing concerns and worries about the issue. At a conference of the California Society of Plastic Surgeons in early 1976, a former president of the society approached Rathjen about the likelihood that leaking silicone gel would migrate to other organs in the human body. Dr. Donald Barker, of Van Nuys, California, suggested that he might do his own tests on the Dow Corning implants— something that immediately raised a red flag for the company. "I think it would be embarrassing for Dow Corning and for any of our research expertise if we find that this type of testing has to be left to a doctor in the field," wrote Rathjen in a memo. "If he were to come up with something which was detrimental, I think we ought to be prepared for it."

Increasingly, plastic surgeons began to believe that silicone leaking from implants played some role in the hardening of the breasts. "I know of at least one loyal Dow Corning customer who believes that our prosthesis bleeds more than other gel prostheses and is considering shifting to a competitive gel product," wrote Chuck Leach, a Dow Corning marketing executive, in 1977. McGhan, even though much smaller than Dow Corning, had already established a study with 55 plastic surgeons to examine the influence of silicone gel implants on capsular contracture. "Several of our customers, looking to us as leaders in the industry, asked me what we were doing, "Leach's memo continued." I assured them, with crossed fingers, that Dow Corning too had an active 'contracture/gel migration' study underway. This apparently satisfied them for the moment, but one of these days they will be asking us for the results of our studies....In my opinion, the black clouds are ominous and should be given more attention." Leach, a straight-laced Dow Corning career veteran with an unsullied reputation, later said the media "misrepresented" his reference to his "crossed fingers." He wasn't lying, Leach insisted. Instead, he meant it as "a sign of hopefulness," claiming that he already knew Dow Corning had studies in progress at the time. Dow Corning said that a study evaluating breast tissue after operations for capsular contracture had been underway at Northwestern University. The study, by Dr. Edward Kaminski was issued two weeks after Leach wrote his memo. It was submitted to the FDA in July of 1991.

Still, the plastic surgeons Leach spoke with were among a growing number who were urging Dow Corning, as the industry leader, to take a more active role in scientific circles to do more research on silicone migration and its effects and to address publicly that and other concerns. But Eldon Frisch, who now headed the Center for Aid to Medical Research, seemed more worried about educating Dow Corning's competition than delving deeper into potential problems with silicone. "I explained that we had tended, to some extent, to avoid these (conferences) since there seemed to be very little to learn by attending and that whenever we gave papers we only encouraged others to become active in this area or in some instances we provided new information which improved the likelihood of competition," wrote Frisch to his colleagues.

Frisch's view, shared by others at Dow Corning, was somewhat surprising, if only because some critical studies of silicone implants, were beginning to surface. At least one doctor, for example, was already publicly discussing the potential for silicone to migrate from the breast to other parts of the body based on his own animal studies. And the issue was beginning to have an impact in the market. Even Rathjen, who urged the task force to push the new product out, expressed worry about it. In mid-1986 he told colleagues, "I have proposed again and again that we must begin an in-depth study of our gel, envelope, and bleed phenomenon. Capsule contracture isn't the only problem. Time is going to run out for us if we don't get underway. Believe me when I tell you that the ASPRS (American Society of Plastic and Reconstructive Surgeons) is also going to begin their own investigation. A committee will be organized and they will come to the manufacturers asking questions. It would certainly be to our advantage to be ready for them."

Colleen's plastic surgeon, Dr. James Baker, who had

received funding from Dow Corning to put together instructional films and videos, began to turn to other suppliers. By this time, Dow Corning's Center for the Aid to Medical Research was winding down. Si Braley's move into Swanson's department had severely limited his contacts with plastic surgeons, and his retirement in 1977 meant that the person who helped to develop the entire industry was no longer there. Many surgeons missed the personal treatment they would often get from Braley. Braley's absence made Dow Corning appear like any other oversized, corporation that becomes unresponsive and hard to deal with. "Dow Corning was a big, bureaucratic institution," says Baker. "They were stodgy. You'd call there and you would be transferred here and there. At Surgitek, you could get the president on the phone immediately. He was receptive to new ideas and new technology." Dow Corning, although still the industry leader, was losing its reputation as an innovator.

*   *   *

Up until the late 1970s, few people other than plastic surgeons and business insiders knew of any problems at all with breast implants. The general media did little to diminish the growing popularity of the operation. Most newspapers and magazines treated breast augmentation as a vain but relatively harmless fascination, a novelty. The women's magazines treated the operation as a way to create a new, happier woman of beauty and sophistication, the kind of slender yet shapely women that commonly appear in the pages of *Vogue* and *Cosmopolitan*. They seemed to suggest a new social reality: Women could look exactly as they wanted to, thanks to the ingenuity of science and the skills of their plastic surgeons. It was as if breast implants were an important achievement of modern civilization.

The first public hint of serious problems did not surface until 1977, when an investigative story on breast enlargement was published by *Ms.*, the feminist magazine created by Gloria

Steinheim. The September issue of *Ms.* contained a revealing, if inflammatory, article under the headline: "A 60% Complication Rate for an Operation You Don't Need."

The exposé, by Marjorie Nashner and Mimi White, told of "infections, deformities, excessive hardness, painful and disfiguring scars, emotional difficulties"—complications that had already been described in medical journals not read by the general public. The writers reported that significant numbers of physicians opposed breast implant surgery because of its unacceptably high incidence of complications. "They point out that in other fields of medicine, operations with such high complication rates are discouraged, except when necessary to save a life or preserve a vital function," *Ms.* reported.

One plastic surgeon, Dr. Dennis Thompson, told the reporters that more than 60 percent of women with implants will develop a problem, the most frequent one being breasts that harden. "Unfortunately, like the victims of rape, most of these patients refuse to come forward," said Dr. John Goin, a plastic surgeon who had placed a notice in *Daily Variety*, hoping to track down women with breast implants for a study he was doing. "There are innumerable disturbed and credulous people who harbor the forlorn hope that an aesthetic operation will produce magical changes in their lives. The merchandising of aesthetic operations...will bring a holocaust of psychological and physical disorders."

The *Ms.* article—accompanied by another on the danger of liquid silicone injections—set off alarms at Dow Corning in Midland, especially because the magazine accused the company of selling what it called "inadequately tested implants." Though offering no details to support its charge, the story did quote yet another plastic surgeon who worried that animal tests weren't sufficient to prove the safety of the devices in human beings. "You cannot compare a test of any implant on a rabbit for 18 months with a breast implant a young woman may have in her body for 30 or 40 years," Dr. David White was quoted as saying. "It would seem that the patients are serving as rabbits for testing these implants."

John Swanson was enlisted to help Melvin E. Nelson,

health care business manager, draft an official response to the magazine story. He read the article with interest, especially since his wife had now had her implants for four and one-half years. It was the first time he had read a negative commentary about breast augmentation and the company's implants. Although the article raised some troubling issues, Swanson thought it failed to provide much documentation to support its charges. He believed the article was sensationalistic and did not connect its allegations to Colleen's implants and the migraine headaches she had begun to have shortly after her surgery. So Swanson had no problem helping to craft a fairly polite letter to the editor that would carry Nelson's signature.

Nelson's first instinct was to write a lengthy, detailed, scientific defense of the implants. He was, after all, analytical by nature, like most of the chemists at Dow Corning. But Swanson assured him that the readers of *Ms.* would be put off by that kind of response. Instead, he helped to draft one of those corporate letters that registers an almost polite objection. The two worked through many drafts, until finally coming up with a reply that actually began by stating that the *Ms.* articles were "interesting and provocative." Ostensibly preferring not to be overly negative, Swanson and Nelson decided not to bring up the assertion that Dow Corning put its first implants on the market without adequate testing.

"While we truly believe our design and materials are the best available, that alone does not prevent the possibility of complications," Nelson stated in the letter. "Dow Corning mammary prostheses are promoted and sold only to the medical profession and never to the general public. Their use for cosmetic or reconstructive surgery is strictly a patient–physician decision. One issue that should always be discussed prior to implant surgery is the formation of scar tissue, which is formed whenever an object is placed in the body. The extent to which scar tissue can become a 'complication' depends on each patient's medical history, her body chemistry, and the surgical procedure used. The article seriously misleads your readers by grossly exaggerating real experience with mammary prostheses."

Even though Swanson thought the *Ms.* piece was mostly hyperbole, he was intrigued enough by the company's position to make at least a small issue of it. What bothered him was the single line in the response that revealed the company's belief that its responsibility for the product ended with the sale of the implants to the doctors. With the exception of medical devices, of course, Dow Corning sold its industrial products to the end user and therefore could take direct responsibility for the product or material it made. With implants, the company asserted that its responsibility ended once the product was sold.

The position troubled Swanson. He believed it was at odds with the code of ethics, which declared, "We will be responsible for the impact of Dow Corning's technology on the environment." The Business Conduct Committee and the company's management at that time defined "technology" as the company's products, and they defined "environment" to include not only the air, earth, and water, but also people. The code, to Swanson's mind, meant that the company would take responsibility for the impact of its products on people. And in his outside talks on ethics he would often say that this single statement was the strongest one in the code.

In truth, Dow Corning's code of conduct was written for an industrial enterprise, not a medical specialty company. Some other medical companies would take a far different approach than Dow Corning. Johnson & Johnson, for example, is guided by its renowned Credo, which clearly spells out the company's responsibilities to the users of its products. Thus, J & J does not hesitate to directly provide end users of its products with specific information via 800 numbers and consumer advertising.

Concerned by what he was beginning to see as a conflict with his own company's code, Swanson decided to get the issue out in the open at a media training seminar he organized for the company's senior management. He had promoted the idea of such sessions for years, hoping to sensitize the company's top executives to potentially embarrassing issues and improve their ability to deal with the media. Though media training had become fashionable, Dow Corning's executives especially needed it. Protected from public scrutiny and accountable only to its two corporate shareholders—Dow Chemical and Corning Inc.—the company grew up without having to grapple with the demands and rigors that commonly face publicly owned corporations. Its management ranks were dominated by chemists and chemical engineers, mostly white males, who were educated in Midwestern universities. As they rose through the ranks in this cloistered environment, few of them worried about their public communications or crisis management skills. Those attributes were not criteria for career advancement at Dow Corning.

Indeed, when Swanson brought in a communications expert in the late 1970s to run the seminars, the consultant was amazed at how insular the company's culture and its executives were. Arnold Zenker, the Boston-based consultant hired to do the media training, would work with the company for more than a decade, into the 1990s. "The culture had created a bored group of executives," says Zenker. "It was not stimulating. They would come into the sessions quiet, and they were counting the days to retirement. It was civil service." Not surprisingly, Zenker found executives ill-prepared to deal effectively with the public. "They were not great communicators, and they were hard to work with because they had no way of putting media training into practice," he says. "It was like working with adolescents at best. They were ingenuous and naive about the media. They were in the middle of cowfields and pastures, isolated from the real world."

Zenker, who has a voice as penetrating and accusatory as Mike Wallace's, is tough, clever, and quick. "In the early years, they were terrified of me," he says. "They weren't used to anyone being brusque or abrasive with them. You could walk through the halls of Dow Corning and never hear a loud voice. You'd think it was a tomb. Everyone was polite. If you shouted at someone, you had no career left at Dow Corning."

So when Zenker, in his very first session in October 1978, gathered all the members of the executive committee in the company's video studio for the first training seminar, there were some curious executives wondering what they would encounter. The studio—then located in the company's original headquarters building across the street from Dow Chemical's sprawling production complex—was a drab room, with a few chairs, a low table, and a plain blue backdrop. Zenker brought in his own video operator, who was ready to zoom in on the fidgeting fingers, moist brows, and—in the case of the company's director of research and development—his bright, white socks.

Swanson, more aware than Zenker of the company's most sensitive issues, wrote questions that explored such touchy issues as the company's virtual monopoly position in silicones and its strategy on acquisitions. None of the executives knew exactly what he would be asked until Zenker posed the questions as directly as he could. Halfway through the session, Zenker finally asked the question that challenged the company's contention that its responsibility for implants ended at the time of their sale to doctors. He turned to the company's vice president in charge of sales and marketing.

At Swanson's direction, Zenker demanded: "Let's talk about silicone breast implants. Dow Corning's marketing strategy apparently dictates that your responsibility stops with the doctor. But let's face it, it's not the doctor who has to live with the bad after effects—a 60 percent complication rate according to *Ms.* magazine. What many people have trouble understanding is that while you [Dow Corning] spend a few million dollars promoting your safe sealants and defoamers to the end user, you don't spend a red cent to give thousands of young women the true facts about implants. And at the same time, warn them about silicone breast injections [sic]. It may represent a small percentage of your sales, but don't you feel some ethical and moral obligation to do more than you are doing?"

Even from the first session, Zenker says he sensed that the company was vulnerable to negative coverage of silicone breast implants. "There was always an awareness that there was a potential media time bomb for silicone breast implants," he recalls. "But they were genuinely pretty ethical folks, and they felt they were doing a service to women who had mastectomies."

Swanson, who attended many of the media training sessions, recalls that the answer to Zenker's question was based on the company's contention that its primary responsibility was to provide implant information to the doctors. It was the plastic surgeons who were responsible for getting that information to their patients. The response would have convinced few watchers of *60 Minutes* or any other news show had any one of these executives ever been questioned by a reporter. Indeed, years later, Robert T. Rylee, then the company's health care business manager, would face a similar question from a real reporter at the local *Midland Daily News.* Rylee said exactly what was said years earlier in the video room. It is the doctor's responsibility to pass that [safety information about breast implants] on to the patients. "We don't know who the patients are."

*   *   *

Even though her clothes fit more comfortably, even though she looked much better in a sweater than ever before, no one knew that Colleen had enhanced her appearance thanks to a Dow Corning product. No one other than her husband and two children knew that she had been a patient, not even the Swansons' friends, parents, or other relatives. Colleen was generally pleased with her new appearance, although she thought her breasts might be slightly bigger than she wanted.

She never flaunted her breasts and she continued to dress conservatively. But Swanson thought her self-esteem had risen immediately after the operation. She did indeed look better. Moreover, she seemed more confident and less shy about her appearance. Never particularly introverted, Colleen had become more outgoing, believed Swanson. "She just seemed to be more social and generally happier," he said. She was also able to find far more clothing that complimented her figure than ever before, making shopping an enjoyable experience at last.

With her new look and their still new marriage, the Swansons seemed like teenagers in love for the first time. They often would have candlelit dinners on the floor in front of the fireplace of their new home, a beautiful Georgian colonial on Bloomfield Drive. She would occasionally accompany him on business trips, sometimes spending a weekend to explore different cities. On most weekends, they'd get into the car and drive a few hours to another Michigan city where Swanson would play golf with his Dow Corning colleagues while Colleen shopped with the other wives, until they met in the evening for dancing and dinner. They traveled together to Myrtle Beach, to St. Augustine, and to the Bahamas to soak up the sun, play still more golf, and enjoy their new life together. Colleen took golf lessons, and they joined the Midland County Club.

The merger of their families proved successful, too. All four children got along well. Swanson's daughters, four-year-old Jolene and eight-year-old Sarah, visited twice a week. During spring break, the Swansons would take them on vacation. Colleen's children, 13-year-old Kathleen and 16-year-old Kelly, were still in school.

For no apparent reason, and certainly none the Swansons could attribute to the implants, Colleen began to suffer from headaches. The pain started gradually, shortly after she received the implants, but over several months built to something far more severe and troubling: migraine headaches that aspirin or simple pain-killers could not relieve. They erupted suddenly and inexplicably. A brain scan failed to show any problems, and the pain would vanish for two weeks or so at a time. But the headaches always returned, the pain becoming excruciating, often localizing in one side of her head. She would get sick to her stomach, unable to eat or sleep. She would sometimes lie in bed moaning, tears streaming from eyes rolled back in her head. All the shades were pulled down to keep out the light, so she could remain hidden in a dark room for three or four days at a time. The pounding became so bad that a doctor would inject her in the hip with pain killers. An oxygen tank was placed by her bedside to ease the stress and anxiety that seemed to overtake her as the pains grew more debilitating. Yet, no doctor could figure out what was wrong.

Then, in 1976, just two years after having her implants installed, she noticed red rashes beginning to appear on her chest, below the armpits and down the rib cage. Soon after, she began to experience pain in her lower back. In 1980 she began working as a dental assistant and the back problems worsened. She went to several doctors who put her through physical therapy, asked her to wear a back brace, and pre-scribed pain killers that made her drowsy. But the pain was unrelenting, even requiring that she be helped out of bed and into cars. After being hospitalized for ten straight days, she quit her job in 1984 on the advice of her physicians.

Still, one ailment seemed to feed into another and yet another. First the migraine headaches, then the rashes, the lower back problems, and, the numbness and pain in both arms and hands. The doctors put her through carpal tunnel tests in 1987, but they proved negative. A biopsy discovered precancerous cells in her uterus so Colleen was scheduled for a uterine freeze, a procedure in which liquid nitrogen is inserted into the organ to destroy all good and bad tissue alike. Shortly after that, she began hemorrhaging from time to time—still with no clues or theory as to why her health was faltering so dramatically.

She would get rashes, sometimes as much as a foot long, in her armpits and down the sides of her body. "I kept thinking I must be allergic to a deodorant so I would switch deodorants and the rashes would come and go," she recalls. Her chest would break out in an unhealthy crimson as if she had been overexposed to the sun. She would blame the detergent she was using in the wash.

Her left shoulder became inexplicably frozen in 1988, requiring extensive physical therapy and regular cortisone shots. It wasn't until a year later, when a doctor manipulated the shoulder in a surgical procedure, that she found some relief. Nonetheless, something was attacking her body, she thought, like a virulent toxin. For the first time, she asked her doctor if her frozen shoulder could have been caused by the silicone in her breasts. It was just a question, not an accusation, because they had gone through every possible explanation for her problems and none of them seemed to fit. The doctor, courteous and brisk, said it was possible and left it at that. She had been selling real estate at the time, and was becoming so fatigued that she could no longer go up and down the steps of the homes listed for sale. One Sunday, she sat silent and exhausted in the real estate office until another broker came in and asked her what was wrong. Colleen broke into tears. "I can't handle this anymore," she cried.

For three to four years, beginning in 1989, she would get a burning pain in the left breast area that felt "like a hot poker." She'd go for a checkup and a mammogram and the doctors could never find anything. "All the tests would come back negative," she says. Her breasts began to harden in the late 1980s, and she felt a constant burning pain in the chest.

Swanson could always read Colleen by her expressive eyes. If she was feeling well, her eyes were alive and bright. If not, her eyes couldn't hide the pain. Increasingly, that is what he saw: disoriented and hurting eyes. Colleen's health problems began to seize control over their life together, severely undermining the daily activities of a once happy and productive existence. Swanson saw it as a gradual, insidious depletion of the quality of their lives.

Wracked by exhaustion and pain, Colleen began to withdraw more and more from life. She began going to bed at 7:30 or 8:30 P.M. instead of 10 or 11. And then it became even earlier, to the point that she was out for the night immediately after dinner. Swanson tried to be patient and conciliatory, but Colleen's illness was beginning to drag him down as well. "There was a time I said to Colleen, 'We really have to take stock and look at our lives and examine what's happened to us. Look,' I said, 'this is not living. The quality of our life has really deteriorated and we've got to find out why.'"

Colleen thought her husband believed the source of many of her problems was in her head, and sometimes Colleen herself wondered. "We would do less and less and less," she remembers. "I had always been a high energy person, and when John would say, 'Let's go do something,' I would pack my bags in five minutes and go. But then I started making excuses because I didn't feel like it. I tried not to let it consume my life, but it became more and more difficult."

Indeed, they had to decline so many invitations for dinner and other events that they became nearly expert at it. "We became very good at making excuses," recalls Swanson. "Our friends would ask us out, but many times we figured out ways to make excuses. We got pretty adept at it. We never said Colleen doesn't feel well or is sick, but we tried to make other excuses."

At one low point, 10 years into her ordeal, she remembers herself slumped in a lawn chair behind their home, silently facing the 14th hole of the Midland Country Club's golf course, in a complete funk. She had found this house, their second home together, when her husband was on a business trip to Europe in the summer of 1986. Colleen called him at 2:30 A.M. in France to tell him about it. She knew he had always wanted to live on the golf course. Almost across the street was the town's impressive library and the Midland Center for the Arts. It was a dream location and a dream house. But now, everything seemed to be slipping from her grasp. "I was thinking to myself we have everything: a lovely home, children, grandchildren. Why am I feeling so bad? I kept thinking I have everything to live for, but I wasn't sure I wanted to live. I had less and less energy. I didn't know if I was fatigued or depressed because I wasn't fulfilling my job as a wife, a mother, a grandmother. We went to fewer social engagements. When I did go, I tried to appear like I had it all together, but I didn't. I had lost all interest in sex. I was starting to go to bed before it got dark and I went right to sleep."

Their life together was falling apart, along with her own health.

"WHY THE HELL ARE WE IN THIS BUSINESS, ANYWAY?"

As Colleen Swanson was beginning to lose more of her energy and more of her life, a San Francisco jury had shocked Dow Corning in 1984 with an unprecedented verdict. After a four-week trial, the jury had returned a $1.7 million verdict in favor of Maria Stern, who once had Dow Corning implants in her chest.

Dow Corning had been sued before by women with breast implants. Most of these cases, however, alleged strict product liability problems and had quietly been settled out of court. The Stern case was the very first to allege that a woman was suffering from systemic, autoimmune disease as a result of silicone.

A once healthy woman who worked for the United States Forest Service, Stern agreed to have implants after she lost her breasts due to a double mastectomy. It wasn't long after she acquired the devices that Stern experienced—as one of her witnesses had put it—"the major hallmarks of human adjuvant disease." Shortly after the rupture of one of her implants, she began to suffer severe weight loss, hair loss, liver dysfunction, and swelling of her lymph nodes, as well as fatigue and weakness. Granulomas—noncancerous lumps or nodules of inflammatory cells—formed where silicone leaked into her body and combined with tissue. Leaking silicone found its way into such sensitive organs as her thyroid gland. After the accessible silicone was removed from Stern's body, some of her most severe immune reactions significantly diminished.

The case attracted surprisingly little attention in the media. Stern's attorneys tried unsuccessfully to get local reporters to cover the trial, but the verdict won no more than a few paragraphs in the San Francisco papers and *The Wall Street Journal.* Swanson couldn't even recall seeing a story on the verdict in the *Midland Daily News.* So few details publicly emerged about the evidence presented in the Stern trial. "I wasn't concerned at that time at all and had little interest in it," Swanson recalls. "There wasn't much talk about it." Corporate gossip simply had it that the case was badly bungled by Dow Corning's legal department and its outside counsel. A few insiders believed that the case should never have gone to trial and could have been settled out of court for a mere fraction of the jury's verdict, with no publicity.

John Swanson also remained firm in his belief that silicone was biologically inert. Like most people at Dow Corning, he didn't take the case seriously at the time. Swanson failed to make a connection between Maria Stern's experience and his wife's health problems.

*   *   *

Even Stern's own attorneys at Hersh and Hersh, a small San Francisco law firm specializing in product liability, initially had some doubts. Until then, the relatively few lawsuits against Dow Corning for its breast implants had resulted in out-of-court settlements for $30,000 to $75,000. Still, Nancy Hersh, whose father Leroy founded the firm, had fashioned a career out of taking obscure cases involving women's health soon after graduating from the University of California's Boalt Hall School of Law in 1970. Nancy Hersh had done some of the earliest legal work on DES (diethylstilbestrol), the drug given to women to prevent miscarriages. The drug was later found to cause vaginal and cervical cancer in thousands of daughters of women who took it in the 1950s and 1960s. Hersh had also worked on product liability cases involving the Dalkon Shield, the birth control device that caused numerous injuries in women. Those cases and her own liberal political leanings left her with what she calls a "healthy, cynical disbelief in the integrity of big corporations."

Stern went to Hersh in February 1982, three months after having her breast implants removed. She had decided to have the implants six years earlier after her physician recommended a mastectomy because of the growth of cystic fibroid tumors in Stern's breasts. Stern, a petite and pretty woman with dark hair and eyes, had the first tumor removed at the age of 23. By 1976, her doctor had excised five grape-sized tumors from her breasts. Though they were noncancerous, Stern's physician was concerned that the tumors could lead to breast cancer. So Stern, who started off fighting fires for the United States Forest Service and ended up as a purchasing agent, agreed to have the mastectomy and the plastic surgery as well. Like Colleen, Stern says her surgeon assured her the implants were safe and minimized any risks that might be associated with the procedure.

Soon after she received her implants, Stern began to experience health problems, ranging from severe fatigue to weight loss. "I lost in excess of 30 pounds," recalls Stern. "I lost 50 percent of my hair. I was losing my ability to see, hear, and touch. My body was shutting down. I was dying. I went to five different doctors, and I couldn't get an answer for what was happening to me."

Sent to Stanford University by one of her physicians, she was examined by Thomas Burns, then a Stanford fellow in rheumatology. He reviewed Stern's medical records and decided to do a search of the medical literature on silicone. Burns discovered an early Japanese paper—a study on silicone injections, not implants—that warned of the potential for silicone to cause health problems and an unpublished Australian paper that confirmed his view that Stern should have her implants removed.

Shortly afterward, Stern's sister-in-law, a lawyer herself,

referred her to Nancy Hersh. "She came to me and wondered if the rupture would serve as the basis of a lawsuit," says Hersh. "I thought probably it was. I looked at Dow Corning's product literature and it essentially said the implants would last a lifetime and would only rupture due to some kind of external trauma. So we filed a lawsuit not knowing what we would find. But my presumption was that we would find something."

At one point, after her implants were taken out, Stern's lymph nodes had been removed. Hersh got the slides of her tissue from that operation and brought them to a pathologist at Pacific Medical Center in San Francisco on the hunch that perhaps silicone had leaked into Stern's lymphatic system. The pathologist, who had testified for Hersh in a previous case, discovered star-like foreign material inside the human tissue. "So now we had a woman with ruptured breast implants that weren't supposed to rupture, and we had silicone in her lymph nodes which were removed because they were enlarged."

Hersh assigned Dan C. Bolton, a young law clerk at the firm who had never worked on a lawsuit before, to work on the Stern case in 1982. Bolton, then 25, was in his last year of law school at nearby Hastings College, where Nancy Hersh taught law as an associate professor. A tall, lean man with brown hair and eyes, he had been attracted to law simply because he loved to argue on behalf of a cause.

When Bolton began the standard paperwork for the case, he had no idea that it would help make his career in law. As part of discovery—the search for documents and witnesses for a case—Bolton filed a generic set of "interrogatories" with Dow Corning. In every product liability suit, it's standard practice to ask for such things as a company's tests to prove a product's safety and effectiveness as well as records of consumer complaints. Most companies then contend that the release of such documents would hurt their competitive position or that the time and money needed to produce the documents amounts to an unreasonable burden on the company.

What quickly amazed Hersh, who would actually try the case, and her young assistant was how adamant Dow Corning was in its refusal to budge on even the smallest issues. "At first, they were completely uncooperative," recalls Bolton. "They just didn't want to produce any of the documents we requested. We made a series of motions to the court to gain access to them. Once the company agreed, it insisted we couldn't copy them. We could take notes from the documents but it would have to see what we were writing down."

So incensed was United States District Court Judge Marilyn Hall Patel at the company's stonewalling that she took the highly unusual step of preventing Dow Corning's attorneys from deposing the plaintiff's experts. It was a serious sanction imposed by the judge because the company employed every tactic imaginable to delay the case and make it more difficult for Stern's lawyers to obtain documents from the company's files. "Our lawyers kept putting everything off, violating motions, refusing to produce documents, and making it very difficult," recalls a former Dow Corning executive. "What they were trying to do is make it so difficult on the plaintiff's lawyers that they would back down. Only the opposite result occurred. It was a great mistake. They pissed off the judge. That is always destructive." Indeed, the judge fined the company at least twice for its refusal to comply with orders by the court. Judge Patel later said the litigation was marked by "an appalling lack of cooperation between the parties, particularly on the part of the defendant, regarding discovery."

The stalling tactics also failed miserably at getting Stern's attorneys to ease up. If anything, the delays gave them reason to think the company was trying to hide something. Bolton and another law clerk, Patricia Szumowski, finally flew to Midland in 1983 to look through the requested materials. Surprisingly, Dow Corning paid for both of them to fly first class. An in-house attorney, John Rigas, was placed in charge of their visit, and on the first day, he took them out to lunch at the Midland Country Club. That afternoon, Rigas locked the pair in a room at the company's corporate headquarters building. "I remember it was a large, cold, dark room," says Bolton. "There must have been 200 boxes of documents in there. The boxes were not labeled. It was all thrown together. But we opened every box and looked through each one, and developed a plan to examine every memo in them."

As the two pored over thousands of internal memos, letters, safety studies, and complaints, they could scarcely believe their eyes. "It was just incredible," recalls Bolton. "It could not have been scripted any better. We found memos that expressed concerns about the lack of long-term testing. We found memos from the company's own marketing reps and salesmen relaying complaints from doctors. I don't think they had any idea of what was in those boxes. They basically collected a lot of documents, stuck them in these boxes, and thought that no one would ever go through them."

Every evening, Bolton would call Nancy Hersh in San Francisco to report yet another damaging discovery in one of the 200 or so boxes. "Some of them I would yank out because I didn't think we ever would see them anymore," says Bolton. During their one-week stay, he and Szumowski photocopied about a dozen of the most incriminating documents they discovered and left requests with Dow Corning for perhaps 1500 more pages of other documents they wanted. By the time they boarded the airplane for their return trip to San Francisco, Bolton felt genuinely excited by the prospect that "we were already beginning to develop a strong case on punitive damages against the company."

Among the most valuable documents were the company's complaint files from plastic surgeons who groused about Dow Corning implants that ruptured in the operating room as they tried to install them in women's breasts. Hersh particularly focused on a series of letters written by a prominent plastic surgeon in Las Vegas, Charles A. Vinnick. In a letter dated September 23, 1981, Vinnick complained about a "failed silicone gel implant" he had taken from a patient. A pathology report showed, according to Vinnick, that the patient suffered "considerable silicone reaction to the extruded material.... I believe this proves the point that 'pure silicone' can cause severe foreign body reactions in susceptible individuals," wrote Vinnick.

Four years later, Vinnick wrote Dow Corning about another patient from whom he had removed a pair of silicone implants. He reported that the gel in a ruptured implant was "terribly runny" while the gel inside the other implant was of "ideal cohesion." The difference led him and some others to believe that when the silicone gel came into contact with tissue fluids and fat the gel's consistency changed. "I feel that your company has both a moral and legal obligation to make this information available through your representatives and in your literature," wrote Vinnick in a September 11, 1985, letter to Dow Corning. "I am loathe to publish my series of cases as I feel that it may open [a] Pandora's Box. I do feel, however, that rapid dissemination of this information is very necessary to protect your company and my colleagues."

But there was more, much more, in the documents Bolton brought back to Hersh. One study on monkeys showed that silicone particles could migrate into other organs of the body. A published article coauthored by none other than Dow Corning's Si Braley on a study of four dogs implanted with miniature silicone breast implants appeared to misrepresent the full findings of the experiment. And there was the "crossed-fingers" memo from marketing executive Chuck Leach, who assured plastic surgeons at a convention that the company had an active study underway to determine whether leaking silicone could migrate to other organs of the body and cause hardness of the breasts.

Surprisingly, despite the highly damaging nature of the documents Bolton discovered in Midland, Dow Corning offered only $75,000 to settle the Stern case before it went to trial. Stern refused the offer. "If they offered something in the low six figures, we might have thought about it," remembers Bolton. "It was the first trial. No one knew how it would play out. We didn't know if the jury would rule in favor of punitive damages. If they were smart, they would have offered us a little more money."

It was a remarkably foolish mistake by the company, given the embarrassing admissions made by Dow Corning scientists, salesmen, and managers in many of the memos discovered by Bolton. But top management was so convinced of the safety of the product that it did not take seriously Stern's claims that the implants had caused her immune problems. "No one at Dow Corning thought this was a serious case," says Robert T. Rylee, II, then vice-president of the company's medical products businesses. "At the time it was going on, I hadn't really followed it. I didn't think it was a big deal. Our in-house counsel was of the opinion that it wasn't a big deal. The medical evidence was such that you had to say it's a bullshit issue."

Ostensibly upset at the failure of its outside legal counsel to convince Judge Patel that it should not have to produce the documents on proprietary grounds, Dow Corning fired the law firm of Sangster and Mannion months before the start of the trial. Sangster and Mannion, which had handled a couple of other breast implant suits for Dow Corning, would never again receive work from the company. In its place, the company hired another San Francisco firm, Low, Ball and Lynch. The firm, whose name prompted much humor from the plaintiff's side, was a general civil and trial practice firm that dabbled in everything from insurance and matrimonial law to estate planning. It was not known as a major player in product liability litigation. The Dow Corning defense was assigned to David B. Lynch, an attorney with over two decades of experience, and Joyce Marie Cram, who had been admitted to the bar seven years earlier, in 1976. Instead of trying to create a better working relationship with Judge Patel, one of their first moves was to file a motion demanding that the judge recuse herself from the trial—an action that hardly endeared Lynch or his client to Patel. "It only made her more angry," says Bolton. "So going into the trial things were not going real well for Dow Corning."

Moreover, Dow Corning's general counsel, Jim Jenkins, had originally assigned a young, relatively inexperienced lawyer in his department, Marcia Marsh, to oversee the case and the outside counsel hired to litigate it. Marsh was a close friend of Jenkins, who served as her mentor. Just weeks before the start of the trial, however, Dow Corning abruptly recalled Marsh to Midland, put her in a new job overseeing trademarks, and replaced her with John Rigas, the attorney who watched over Bolton when he was shuffling through the company's papers. Rigas, who was still relatively new to the company, had little time to prepare for the Stern case.

When the trial began, one of the key issues was the question of informed consent. Was Stern clearly informed of the risks she was taking when she agreed to have implants? Like Colleen Swanson, Stern had based her decision to have the implants in large part on a congenial Dow Corning document: "Facts You Should Know About Your New Look." Filled with the promise of a better self-image and a more attractive body, the brochure said nothing about the likelihood that small amounts of silicone would leak into the body, or the possibility that implants could rupture, spilling silicone into other parts of the body. It said nothing about complications such as enlarged lymph nodes, scar formation, inflammation, or other problems that could occur when gel leaked from an implant. It said nothing about the potential for silicone to cause systemic illness with joint pain, fatigue, fever, body rashes, weight loss, skin lesions, and other symptoms. And it largely minimized the most common problems that women often experienced with implants—capsular contracture due to the formation of scar tissue around the implants. Instead, the brochure listed a series of commonly asked questions with reassuring answers.

"How long will the mammary prosthesis last?"

"Based upon laboratory findings, together with human experience to date, one would expect that the mammary prosthesis would last for a natural lifetime. However, since no mammary prosthesis has been implanted for a full life span, it is impossible to give an unequivocal answer."

"Can I expect any problems with my breasts following mammary augmentation?"

"While thousands of women have mammary augmentation operations done annually without any adverse reactions, no surgical procedure is a success every time, and each person's reactions to surgery and implantation can be different. Occasional complaints of excessive breast firmness and/or discomfort caused by fibrous capsule formation and shrinkage have necessitated surgical correction and have been noted in the medical literature."

The brochure—read by hundreds of thousands of women contemplating implant surgery—had been put together by a Dow Corning public relations man, Bob Emmons, and a Chicago-based advertising agency, Siber-McIntyre. The suggestion that implants would last a person's lifetime was based on no scientific report or field study, but on the beliefs of the company's scientists and engineers. "It's what we believed at the time," recalls Emmons, who now owns a medical supply company in Atlanta. "We were naive. But there was no conspiracy [for misleading people]. We were too dumb to conspire. Our engineers and scientists told us silicone was completely inert, and women would look good with them for the rest of their lives."

At Stern's trial, the company's optimistic brochure would cause it considerable trouble. Some of the most riveting testimony on this point came from Marc A. Lappe, then an adjunct associate professor at the University of California at Berkeley's School of Public Health. Lappe, an expert on the subject of informed consent, was asked by Hersh to examine many of the documents unearthed by Bolton so that he could be a witness in the case. He was sent four boxes full of Dow Corning memos and studies to review in advance of the trial.

Reviewing the "New Look" brochure against many biosafety studies in the boxes, Lappe quickly came to the conclusion that no woman who decided to have implants based on the company's literature was fully aware of the risks she was taking because Dow Corning failed to disclose such risks. "They [the brochures] were inaccurate," he claims. "They were incomplete, and they were deceptive." Lappe concluded that Dow Corning had, in effect, conducted a 30-year "medical experiment" on a million or more women who had not been able to make an informed choice because all of the information about the safety of silicone implants had not been made available to them.

It was while Lappe was on the stand that he was asked to

examine the article coauthored by Si Braley, Swanson's old friend, published in 1973 in a journal called *Medical Instrumentation*. In describing the findings of the study in which four dogs were implanted with miniature silicone breast implants, Braley and his coauthor, Gordon Robertson, had largely reported the results of the two-year study at its six-month mark—even though the article was published after the study's completion. At six months, the authors reported there was some minor inflammation in some of the dogs—but nothing unusual. Joyce Cram, the outside counsel who tried the case for Dow Corning, wanted to use the document, among others, to show that the company had properly tested the implants and they were safe.

Asked to comment on the study, Lappe recalled that he had seen the raw data upon which the article was based among the more than 4000 pages he had examined in the four boxes he was sent. Something wasn't right, Lappe thought, but he couldn't put his finger on it. It was nearing the end of the day so Judge Patel permitted his testimony to be concluded the following morning.

"I didn't get much sleep that night," Lappe recalls. "Both the left and right sides of my brain were battling as to where I had seen this information. I finally went to sleep, but at four in the morning, something woke me up. I went downstairs and pulled out the original animal data. What the data showed was that while these animals were all right at six months, at two years one had died and the other three had varying degrees of very severe chronic inflammation. These animals did not do well with their implantable devices." Indeed, besides the one death, two dogs suffered chronic inflammation, thyroiditis, autoimmune response, and spots on the spleen.

Back on the stand, Lappe had begun to testify about his findings when he was interrupted by Dow Corning's attorney, who objected to Lappe's remarks on the grounds that such details about the study had not been discovered during the course of his three-day deposition and were therefore inadmissible. Judge Patel, however, began to question the witness herself, until she asked to see the documents on the study that both Lappe and the company's attorneys had brought into the court. The identifying numbers on the dogs were different on the two sets of documents. "My copy only had the last two digits of the four numbers identifying each dog," says Lappe. "Their copy had all four digits." It looked as if Dow Corning had altered the data to make it more difficult for outsiders to get at the full two-year results of the study. It was a key reason, believes Hersh, that the jury would later find the company guilty of fraud.

Right from the start, Nancy Hersh felt confident she was winning every day she left the courtroom. "I don't think they tried the case properly because they were so arrogant and confident they were going to win," says Hersh. "Maybe they underestimated me and our witnesses. But the trial was one great day after another. You should feel good at the end of the day when you put your case on. But when you feel great at the end of the day when they are putting their case on, you know you're winning big." Indeed, at one point during the trial the company sought to settle the case for $150,000, but Hersh refused.

The case brought Si Braley, by then retired, Art Rathjen, and other Dow Corning managers into the courtroom to testify. Dow Corning's experts, however, were generally poorly prepared and disorganized. "They were truly awful," says Bolton. "They went along with us up to a certain point, acknowledging that implants could rupture, that silicone could bleed from the implant and migrate to other parts of the body. But they were also hostile and openly combative." One Dow Corning scientist, recalls Bolton, suggested that Stern had to be suffering from some kind of mental disease because she had the audacity to think her immune problems were caused by silicone.

Moreover, Dow's witnesses opposed a sympathetic plaintiff in Stern. She was married with three children. She had not had implants for cosmetic reasons, so the jury could hardly question her decision to have the surgery. Stern also was obviously ill. Her weight had fallen to 87 pounds from 110, and she sometimes walked into the courtroom with a cane. Yet, Stern recalls, Dow Corning's attorneys suggested her health problems were caused by anything but silicone, from liver disease to tuberculosis. At one point, she says, defense counsel suggested she was an IV-drug user. Dow Corning's lawyers even tried to prevent her husband from being in the courtroom when she was scheduled to testify in the case.

Such tactics backfired severely. "They never took the case seriously," says Bolton. "Historically, the most they ever paid on an implant case was maybe $30,000 to $75,000 to settle. It was not a big deal to them because they had never paid much, and no one had ever contended in a lawsuit that an immune disease was caused by silicone."

In awarding Stern $211,000 in compensatory damages and $1.5 million in punitive damages—exactly what Hersh had asked for in a punitive award—the jury found that Dow Corning was guilty of selling a poorly designed product with a manufacturing defect in breech of the warranty implied by its "New Look" brochure. The jury found Dow Corning guilty of fraud, believes Hersh, because the company's internal memos and studies suggested far more risks than were revealed in its brochure.

In a post-trial order, Judge Patel called some of the motions filed by Dow Corning's attorneys to undermine the jury's decision "absurd" and "frivolous." "There was substantial evidence before the jury of defendant's knowledge of the inadequacy of its testing and knowledge of rupture and gel bleed," Patel wrote. "There was also substantial evidence of the probable injurious consequences and a conscious, willful failure to inform the consumer." She called the company's behavior "highly reprehensible."

Shortly after the verdict, the case came up for a brief discussion at Dow Corning's board of directors meeting in Midland.

"Why in the hell are we in this business, anyway?" asked Paul Orrefice, then chief executive of Dow Chemical.

Rylee told him the company was making implants mainly to help women who lost their breasts to cancer and to help other women restore their self-esteem by looking more normal. "We should stay in the business from an ethical standpoint," Rylee said. "We have a moral obligation to support the doctors who are treating breast cancer patients. We certainly aren't making much money being in this business."

"Are we going to have much more of this in the future?" asked Orrefice, obviously concerned about the company's future exposure to additional lawsuits.

"It was a case of first impressions," insisted Rylee. "I do not think that the science in any way supported the verdict. I don't think there will be many more of these cases. The legal department feels the same way. They believe this case is an aberration."

Two decades later, recalling the board meeting at which Orrefice asked his incisive questions, Rylee would admit: "With 20-20 hindsight, I was wrong as hell."

Dow Corning appealed the Stern decision and lost, and then appealed again. Before the final ruling could be reached by the Superior Court, the company offered Stern an undisclosed settlement in 1987 that included a protective order that kept all of the documents in the case from being made public and bound every expert witness at the trial to secrecy. She accepted the deal.

Meanwhile, Rylee oversaw an extensive rewrite of the company's package inserts that more fully informed patients of the risks they undertook in having implants. After 1985, the company's package literature described 18 possible "adverse reactions and complications" ranging from breast and nipple inflammations and skin sloughing to immune responses—many of the symptoms from which Colleen Swanson was now suffering.

For 22 years, from the time Dow Corning first began selling silicone implants until the Stern verdict, information warning women of these risks had never been made available. And even in the aftermath of the Stern decision, women getting implants had to rely on their plastic surgeons to fully disclose the potential complications. The reason: Dow Corning was unwilling to provide such details directly to the end users of the devices. The company's asserted responsibility still stopped with the sale of the implants to its direct customers—

the plastic surgeons who were paying about $220 for a pair of Dow Corning implants and charging their patients up to $4000 each for a quick and relatively easy operation. One company official figured that more than 6 of every 10 plastic surgeons failed to inform patients of the full risks of the operation.

SILICONE CRITICS

After a long day of meetings and in-basket memos, John Swanson returned home one evening in late 1990 to hear Colleen accuse Dow Corning of selling an unsafe product and causing the illnesses that had been plaguing her for years. Her daughter, Kathy, had called from Santa Maria, California, earlier in the day after viewing a Geraldo Rivera program about the dangers of silicone breast implants. The show featured several women who had health problems remarkably similar to her mother's and attributed them to their silicone breast implants.

"Mom," Kathy said, "I think I know what's wrong with you."

"Well, what do you mean?" asked Colleen, surprised by the call.

"I just saw this woman on television out here. She has all of your symptoms and she has Dow Corning implants. She's just a classic case of what you're going through."

The woman Kathy was referring to turned out to be Kathleen Anneken, a co-founder of a self-help group called the Command Trust Network and a person who would later play a profound role in Colleen Swanson's life.

It was as if the sun had finally broken through a cloudy sky. For years, doctors had found no physical reason for her many symptoms and problems. Though Swanson had repeatedly assured her he didn't believe that she was imagining her illnesses, Colleen herself had wondered if it was all in her head. Suddenly, she heard a plausible reason for her unexplainable decline. "Every doctor I visited kept saying 'I know there is something wrong with you, but I just don't know what it is,'" she recalls. "After my daughter's call, there wasn't a doubt in my mind that that was it. The symptoms were exactly the same."

For the rest of the day, Colleen resisted any temptation to call her husband at work. She simply allowed the revelation to sink into her consciousness as her mind swung from "I've got to find out what's causing this" to "I think I know what's causing it." If the implants were leaking silicone into her body and the chemical was causing all or most of her problems, she wanted the implants out immediately. If it meant that she would be flat-chested for the rest of her life, she didn't care—as long as she could be given a chance to recover and lead a more normal life again.

What made it worse, of course, was that there had never been a compelling reason to have the implant surgery. She had chosen to have it to improve her appearance, to make her clothes fit better, to be perfect for John Swanson. But it was never absolutely necessary. Colleen would not have done it if she had been even remotely aware of the possible problems. She could only remember all the assurances from Si Braley and from James Baker. But it was a decision she had made and now she knew it was destroying her life, making her and her husband's life together a nightmare.

Whom could she turn to for help? Certainly no one in Midland, she thought. The doctors in town were unlikely to recognize or understand that silicone—a substance responsible for a good deal of the area's affluence and prosperity—could cause so many health problems. Perhaps that was why no one suggested that her implants could have been the source of her illnesses. Why didn't Dow Corning or Dr. Baker or even her husband inform her of the risks? Did they know the hell that breast implants could cause? What would her husband say and think when she told him? Would he think she was grasping at straws? The hours in that day passed swiftly for Colleen, filled with questions that had few answers.

For John Swanson, arriving home after a day's work, her accusation was like a hard punch to the gut. After all, he had played a role in assuring his wife the devices were safe. Like everyone else in little Midland, he thoroughly believed the company line that silicone was an inert substance, harmless and uniquely suited for use in the human body. He had no reason not to believe it. Yet now his own wife was accusing his company of knowingly selling a product that could cause serious health problems.

For nearly 25 years, he had enjoyed a challenging and fulfilling career with a company he believed in. Over the past 15 of those years, he had evolved into Dow Corning's Mr. Ethics. And now the most important person in his life was alleging that Dow Corning had behaved unethically. He wished he could refute his wife's accusations, but he couldn't. If the implants were the cause of her problems, he thought, Dow Corning could not have known of the risks. If it knew, the company would have made full disclosure to women to allow them to make informed decisions about the implants. Swanson could be sympathetic to her charges, but he couldn't agree that silicone had caused her illnesses through the years.

"John," she insisted, "I really think this could be the problem."

"If that's the case," he said, "our lives will be turned upside-down. I'm certain the company will never consider silicone to be a health problem."

"That may be," she countered, "but I can tell you right now they're coming out. At this point, all I care about is living."

They stayed up nearly the entire night, discussing the possibility that the company to which Swanson had devoted his life had somehow betrayed his wife and hundreds of thousands of other women. What would they do now? How would they handle this?

Their primary concern was how to find a reliable and competent doctor they could trust. None of the Midland physicians who treated Colleen had ever once suggested that her implants could be the cause of her health problems. The Swansons now believed that they could not find help in Midland. The community had an adequate hospital and better-than-average doctors and specialists. But Midland was, after all, the silicone capital of the world. It was a gossipy town, and the Swansons knew that there was a real possibility that even a cursory discussion of Colleen's suspected problems with Dow Corning's implants could quickly spread and get back to Swanson's colleagues at headquarters.

Besides, neither of them believed that the doctors in Dow Corning's home community knew enough—or had even the willingness to know enough—about silicone-related illnesses. "We knew we had to get out of Midland to get proper treatment," says Colleen. "We had to leave here because of John's job, and because the doctors in Midland all have Dow Corning patients. They weren't about to step on Dow Corning's toes. It meant that we had to get out of this provincial place we lived in."

Colleen was already sure that the removal of her implants would be far more expensive than the original procedure. "If insurance is going to be a hassle with Dow Corning, let's just forgo it," she told Swanson. "I won't have my health be dependent on Dow Corning's insurance. I'd rather cash in an IRA. We'll have it done, one way or another, away from here so no one here will have to know."

Swanson wasn't so sure. On the basis of one television program and a phone call, Colleen was ready to undergo serious surgery, much more difficult and painful than the operation to put the implants into her breasts. And he could not accept that Dow Corning knew it was selling a product that could hurt someone. "There was no rational or documentable reason to believe it," he says. "Intellectually, I knew where she was coming from; the pains were real, not in her head. But there were all the other nonemotional factors that played into it, too. We had built a good life in Midland and now suddenly all of it—friends, career—was at stake."

Swanson knew that the problem, unlike a 24-hour virus, would not go away. It was unavoidable—at work or at home. At work, he could not help but wonder how much or how little anyone around him knew about the problem. At home, he had to be sympathetic to his wife's illness and her charges against his company. Why hadn't the company's own ethics program— in which he had invested so much of himself—uncovered signs that there was a problem with the devices? Did the company perform adequate testing to insure the product's safety? Was it conceivable that Dow Corning and its executives, including several of his closest friends, had knowingly sold a dangerous product for decades?

Swanson didn't know the answers, and he wasn't yet sure how to react to Colleen's charges—as a husband or as an executive of Dow Corning. "I was in between," he recalls. "I was trying to figure it out. Because I was part of the culture at Dow Corning that led me to believe that these materials are inert and safe and I still was not convinced, even though I'm seeing more and more reason in her case to explore it. We tried everything else. But I really wanted to believe the company."

What Swanson believed, at least during the long hours of that night, didn't mean all that much to Colleen. That evening, she wasn't concerned about his career, their friends, or their life in the close-knit community that sometimes felt like a subdivision of Dow and Dow Corning. She knew her husband was conflicted, trying to be understanding, yet fearful of how her accusations might alter their life together. "I know he wanted what was best for me," recalls Colleen. "His concern was his loyalty to the company and his loyalty to me, plus he's the one who took me to get it done. He did not ask me to have it done. It was my own decision. But I didn't know there was such a thing as implants until I married John. I had no idea. That night was terrible. It was as if our life changed overnight, just absolutely overnight. But I knew one thing for sure: I just wanted them out and I wanted to get well."

*   *   *

After John Swanson reported to work the next morning on only a few hours of sleep, Colleen sat by the telephone and began calling—everyone she could. She spoke to plastic surgeons all over the country, from as close as Saginaw, Michigan, to as far away as Atlanta, Georgia. None of them would agree that her implants were the cause of any of her illnesses. If she wanted to be explanted, they would do it—only if she agreed to have a replacement set put into her chest. Some suggested she see a psychiatrist. One warned her that she would never be able to live with herself if she had the implants removed. Then, she called Kathleen W. Anneken, whose name had come up on the television program Kathy had seen in California.

If Dow Corning had an enemies list, Anneken would have been near the very top of it. Executives privately called her a crazy radical making unsubstantiated charges. Plastic surgeons thought of her as a reckless gadfly, eager to stir up unnecessary anxiety among women with implants. A Covington, Kentucky, housewife-turned-activist, she had had five breast implant surgeries before having the implants removed for good in October 1989. Frustrated by her experiences and hoping to find other women to share her concerns, Anneken, a registered nurse, had listed herself as the head of a national self-help group called Command Trust Network ("Command" standing for cosmetic operation mishaps), which was founded in May 1988.

As diminutive and thin as Colleen, Anneken, too, had decided to get implants to improve her appearance and her self-esteem. She had always been small-chested and troubled by it, even as a shy and quiet student at a Catholic high school. It wasn't until 1972, when she was 26 years old, however, that she read an article in the *Cincinnati Enquirer* on plastic surgery.

"Look, honey," she said to her husband, Dave, "they're selling body parts now. Do we have enough money to do my breasts?"

"You must be joking," her husband responded.

But it wasn't a joke to her. A year earlier, she had been in a serious car accident that put her in an intensive care unit with a collapsed lung and two broken ribs. While the nurses bathed her, she had overheard an uncomplimentary comment about her body that would humiliate her. "For someone who is so small, she has fat legs," one nurse said. Recalls Anneken, "I thought that at least my legs won't look so bad if I had something up top to go with them."

Within days, she had made an appointment to see a local plastic surgeon who said he could do the operation for $1200. "That was nothing, especially to look like someone else," Anneken says. But when she awoke from the surgery performed under general anesthesia at a hospital near her home, she became hysterical. "They were a mess," says Anneken. "The implants were solid as rocks. They were too big. They made me into a size D from a double-A. And they came up to my collarbone. They were so high that my nipples hung off the bottom of the implants pointing straight down.

"No one warned me about this. Yet when I got upset, they called in a psychiatrist and they kept me in the hospital for four days. I was upset because none of this looked normal, and there was no way that anyone would be fooled that they were natural. They said, 'Don't worry. They'll descend. They'll get soft.' I wanted them out the day they went in." Eventually, her breasts would develop ridges like corduroy fabric. She would smooth the ridges out, but they would slowly reappear, often with a slight popping sound.

A year and eight months later, the surgeon finally agreed to take them out and put in a new pair of silicone replacements. After her second operation, she still was too big—a C cup — but the implants looked and felt more natural than before. They remained in her chest until 1986, when she began doing commentary for local fashion shows and some commercial modeling on television. "Unfortunately, I should not have gotten into a business where what you looked like was very important. Here I am in this store-bought chest that now looks abominable. My second implants had become unusually hard, but the major problem was that they were still too big for my body. I decided I'm going to have them fixed."

A third surgery was scheduled, but she wound up with implants that were slightly larger than the ones removed. Within a couple of weeks, one implant began to migrate into her left armpit whenever she lay down. Even worse, the surgeon installed the implants behind her chest muscles—an increasingly popular technique among plastic surgeons at the time. "Besides having implants that were too big, I couldn't do anything with my arms," she recalls. "I lost a lot of strength that my chest muscles provided. My shoulders were hurting. I said, 'Here we go again.'"

What made the experience even more maddening was her surgeon's reaction to her complaints. "He would sit down and say, 'Are you sure you're not having problems at home?'" says Anneken. "And then I would burst into tears. I thought how am I going to tell this guy again and again that the implants weren't right? The doctors turn you into an idiot. And then you go out to your car and you can hardly drive home."

In August of 1987, Anneken went through the operation —for the fourth time. Smaller implants—about 140 cc with a broad base and a flat profile—were ordered, but they arrived in the wrong size—160 cc with a narrow base and a higher profile. "By the time I found out the wrong implants came in, I was in a paper gown on a paper sheet for my fourth surgery. I didn't know how to get out of this mess. I came out looking like I had volcanoes on my chest. That's when I started talking about just having the implants out for good." Within two months, however, one implant had ruptured and she began developing lower joint pains. The doctor had to aspirate blood out of a pocket in her breast. So the plastic surgeon cut her open yet again to replace one of the implants he had put into her only two months earlier.

Baffled by all her trouble, Anneken began to wonder how many other women had similar problems. A month after starting her support group, she saw an article in *Ms.* magazine by a Beverly Hills, California, writer who also had multiple problems with breast implant surgery. Unlike Anneken, Sybil Niden Goldrich had lost both her breasts to cancer in 1983. Before getting implants, she had interviewed four plastic surgeons, read every article on the subject she could find, and even looked through several medical books. Goldrich chose silicone implants because, she was advised, it was the simplest and least traumatic option available to her. Or so she thought.

The implants hardened, became misshapen, and changed position so that they never matched, and all efforts to create a nipple and areola on her breasts caused infection and decay of the skin. At one point, the implants nearly passed through the weakened skin on her chest and out of her body and had to be surgically removed. "Nothing in my research suggested that this 'simple' procedure would turn into five operations, over a period of 10 months, requiring more than 15 hours under anesthesia and countless days of pain and discomfort," she wrote.

Her problems led her to conduct an extensive search for answers. Her husband, James, a doctor, read all the medical articles on silicone they could find. He would highlight the key passages in yellow for her to digest. Goldrich wrote a book about her problems tentatively called *A Whole Body, A Whole Life*, but could not find a publisher for the work. "I had thought my problems were caused by advanced cancer," she says. "It turned out the problems were caused by my implants. Yet, no one believed my story for the longest time."

Ultimately, Goldrich's breasts were restored not by implants but by a transverse abdominal island flap, an intricate operation that uses a patient's own abdominal tissue to recreate the missing breasts. Even so, her traumatic experience with implants left another mark on her. Five years after her first surgery in 1983, silicone was found in her uterus, ovaries, and liver.

Goldrich finally made her story public in *Ms.* magazine in June 1988. Her problems with implants prompted her to do far more research on the topic and what she discovered troubled her. Goldrich found out, for example, that most plastic surgeons defined a failed implant as one literally damaged in manufacturing. To a patient, however, a failed implant is one that causes pain or discomfort or leads to an additional surgery to replace the original device. Using this latter definition, the estimates for failure were much higher than any reported by either the plastic surgeons or the manufacturers. Goldrich unearthed an article by a doctor in the February 1987 issue of *Annals of Plastic Surgery* that estimated that nearly 50 percent of implants after mastectomies required replacement.

After reading her story, Kathleen Anneken wrote a letter to

Goldrich in care of *Ms.* magazine. The two subsequently spoke by telephone. Almost immediately, the two struck up a lively conversation that led to their partnership as co-founders of Command Trust Network in late 1988. The idea was to link implanted women with one another so they could sort through their problems together and to create and distribute consumer information on implants that advised women what kinds of questions they should ask of plastic surgeons before undergoing the operation.

At first, they seemed an unlikely duo. Goldrich was a New Yorker transplanted to California. A professional writer who had also produced television commercials and industrial films, she would probably never have considered getting implants had she not lost her breasts to cancer. She would have thought it frivolous and vain. Anneken, a registered nurse, initially had no qualms about cosmetic surgery and did little research before allowing a surgeon to operate on her. "We were the odd couple," recalls Goldrich. I don't smoke. She does. She is thin. I am overweight. Kathleen is neat and compulsive. My desk looks like World War III. But it wasn't long before we began to finish each other's sentences. We were of one mind, with the same reasonable focus."

Initially, however, both of them were somewhat skeptical of the person on the other end of the telephone. "We were both scared of each other at first," says Anneken. "She didn't know who I was when I called. She might have thought I was a Kentucky hillbilly who wanted to march on Washington. I was worried that Sybil, though she could write a good article, would be too angry to stay cool. But what I can't do, she can, and vice versa. I'm a registered nurse, married to a public accountant. She's a writer, married to a doctor, and has a daughter who is an attorney. We had access to all the skills we needed for Command Trust."

Goldrich helped Anneken through her decision to have the implants taken out for good by a cancer surgeon in Tampa, Florida in October 1989. Even that was an ordeal—Anneken visited eight different doctors in Kentucky, Ohio, Georgia, and Florida, before locating one who agreed to do the operation without replacing the implants. "Many doctors didn't want to do it because they didn't want to deal with any depression their patients might have after losing their breasts," she says.

Anneken and Goldrich, who would finally meet each other in person at an FDA hearing in March 1989, soon began publishing a newsletter and fielding telephone calls from other women with similar problems. "I believed that I would hear from go-go dancers and prostitutes," Anneken says. "Yet every single woman who contacted me has been an enterprising housewife or in business for herself, usually in visually oriented fields, people who like the way things look. These are intelligent, productive members of our society."

In the first year, 1988, Anneken received no more than three calls from women with implants. Then, in January 1989, she heard from three women who all complained that silicone implants had caused them numerous health problems, including auto-immune system disorders. It wasn't until Anneken flew to New York to appear on a Geraldo Rivera show dedicated to implants in March 1989 that Command Trust began to consume more and more of her time. The Rivera show appearance alone attracted 300 letters in just a few days.

The issue was beginning to attract more media attention in 1989 after an FDA staffer leaked a 1987 Dow Corning study to Public Citizen Health Research Group, a Washington, D.C.–based consumer lobby founded by Ralph Nader. The study showed "an increased incidence of fibrosarcomas at the implant site." Immediately, Dr. Sidney Wolfe, director of the Nader research group, held a news conference to report the study and then sued the FDA to release the results of all the safety studies on silicone gel Dow Corning provided to the agency. Previously, Wolfe's group had unsuccessfully petitioned the FDA to ban silicone breast implants on the grounds that they could cause allergic reactions, tissue swelling, and damage to internal organs.

Both Anneken and Goldrich—working behind the scenes—proved tenacious and articulate adversaries of the implant manufacturers and the plastic surgeons. They regularly wrote letters to Washington regulators and politicians to demand that the FDA further examine the devices. And they continually urged their members to do the same, providing addresses and phone numbers of key policymakers from FDA Chairman David A. Kessler to Representa-tive Ted Weiss, a New York liberal Democrat whose subcommittee held hearings on the safety of implants. They helped talk show hosts find women willing to go public with their implant problems. Anneken even became a nonvoting member of the Food and Drug Administration's advisory panel on implants, while Goldrich managed to get herself on another FDA committee to create an informed consent brochure on implants.

It wasn't until late November, however, that the pair received a big media break. The Public Citizen lawsuit filed a year earlier resulted in a victory when, on November 27, 1990, a federal judge ordered the FDA to release the results of two decades worth of Dow Corning studies on silicone along with a list of complaints about the product. United States District Court Judge Stanley Sporkin, moreover, scolded Dow Corning for preventing him from hearing the testimony of expert witnesses familiar with the animal studies. These witnesses had been hired by attorneys in product liability suits the company had settled out of court. In every instance, Dow Corning had won secrecy orders to prevent the testimony from leaking out to the public. Sporkin called the company's behavior "particularly troubling" and then chastised the FDA for its "ineptness" in dealing with Dow Corning and other implant makers. The lawsuit victory prompted a television producer for Connie Chung's *Face to Face* news program on CBS to call Anneken. Chung apparently wanted to do a segment on whether implants caused breast cancer.

"That is going to be a short show," retorted Anneken. "What are you going to say? We don't know the answer yet. It will take 30 years of additional studies to tell. What you ought to look into are all the problems women have after they get implants." Anneken supplied the show with the names of people who had called her over the previous months with complaints and sent the producer articles on the topic, too.

Rather than breast cancer, the program focused on possible links between silicone leakage from breast implants and autoimmune-system diseases such as lupus. It was a milestone of sorts because it was the first time on national television that a medical authority, Dr. Douglas Shanklin, a University of Tennessee pathologist, put the issue Dow Corning most feared out in front: "Silicone gets right into the heart of the immune system," he said.

After the segment aired on December 10, 1990, with a short appearance by Goldrich, the Command Trust Network was swamped with 1000 telephone calls in one week—even though Anneken's number wasn't given out on the air. "We would call each other crying," recalls Goldrich, "because we didn't know what to do." All across the country, women with breast implants were calling their plastic surgeons—even though the show largely focused on polyurethane-coated silicone implants, yet another version of the products. Dr. James Baker—Colleen's plastic surgeon—even had one patient cancel a scheduled breast implant operation after the TV broadcast.

At Command Trust Network, Anneken thought the phone would never stop ringing. She drafted her son and his girlfriend to help with the calls. She installed an answering machine, converted two upstairs rooms of her home to the effort, and spent 12 to 14 hours a day on the phone. Amidst the blitz of telephone calls that followed the Chung show, Anneken had one of the most memorable conversations she would ever have with a desperate silicone victim who called during a busy weekday in December 1990.

*   *   *

As soon as Anneken picked up the phone in her Kentucky home, Colleen told the consumer activist that her husband worked for Dow Corning.

"Oh my God," said Anneken, "you're kidding."

"No, I'm not. This makes my situation even worse."

Anneken, who had already spoken to hundreds of implanted women with problems, says she wasn't shocked by Colleen's call. At first, she thought the caller was a little too trusting with a total stranger on the phone. Then, she wondered if the telephone call was some kind of setup or ploy by Dow Corning to find out what she and Sybil Goldrich were up to. But from the desperation in the voice on the telephone, Anneken surmised that Colleen had to be telling the truth.

"Who can I go to?" Colleen asked her. "I can't go to anybody around here. I can't go to anybody in this state. What am I going to do?"

Anneken shared her own troubles with implants and then gave Colleen the names of a couple of surgeons who do explantations—neither of them in Michigan. The phone call from a wife of a Dow Corning executive—the first, and, as far as she knows, the only one she ever received—genuinely excited Anneken. She thought that if there were more Colleens out there, wives of Dow Corning managers and executives or Dow Corning employees with implants themselves, maybe the company would abandon its defensive posture and begin to help the victims.

For Colleen, the implant activist became a godsend. "I was relieved to have a woman who understood my problem to talk to," she recalls. "She was the first person I ever talked to with implants and with some of the same symptoms I had. On one hand, it was encouraging. On the other, I was getting very scared because now that I knew the cause of my problem, I wondered what we were going to do about it and how it would affect my life. After talking to her for five minutes, I felt as if we had a common bond."

Still, the Swansons wrestled with the idea that Colleen should have her implants out. "I knew that removing the implants was a much more difficult and dangerous operation than putting them in," says Swanson. "So it was not a surgery to go into lightly. You really had to be very sure. In her body and in her mind, she was sure. My role was to make very sure we knew what we were about to do."

Although John Swanson was by now suspicious, he still wasn't entirely convinced that the implants were the cause of

Colleen's deteriorating health. He also wasn't sure that having them out would guarantee the return of her health. Indeed, another complicated surgery might worsen her condition and deal a tremendous blow to her self-esteem because she would be left without breasts. Bit by bit, however, Swanson was coming round to the realization that the implants had to be the source of her health problems. "It was almost by process of elimination that I came to believe it, because she had gone through almost every conceivable test," he remembers. "It wasn't until every possibility was exhausted that I thought maybe, just maybe, it's the silicone. And even after the rational mind said, 'Yeah, maybe there is something there,' the heart and soul would say, because of the company, 'It just can't be.' I was just pulled in two diametrically opposite directions. But more and more, there was nothing else left. It had to be. Finally, I had to admit it. It was hard for both of us to come to that conclusion."

What would bring him closer to that conclusion was an unusual event at work, an unexpected complaint of an ethics violation that would land on his desk. It would shake all his faith in his employer and make him question the morality and the ethics of the company where he had spent more than two decades.

AN ETHICAL ISSUE

Just five days before Christmas in 1990, Swanson opened up a "For Addressee Only" interoffice envelope on his desk and found a shocking memo inside. The document alleged that two company executives were trying to destroy internal reports that showed far higher complication rates for silicone breast implants than the company had ever publicly acknowledged. These were serious allegations, with profound implications, no matter what the circumstances. But for Swanson, there was a personal dimension to the charges because his own wife be-lieved his company was guilty of fraud.

What made the memo all the more startling was that it came from Charles F. Dillon, the company's medical director. Dillon—a very tall man, probably six-foot-four, with reddish hair—had an impeccable reputation inside the company. Like Swanson himself, Dillon was not the type of person to make unfounded charges. Yet, here he was asking the company's Business Conduct Committee to investigate what Dillon termed "a violation of corporate, professional, and commonly accepted business ethics."

As Swanson read the full memo, he could scarcely believe his eyes. It said:

> The specific incident occurred on Friday, December 14 at 5:15 P.M. Greg Thiess, a senior litigation attorney in the corporate legal department approached Mary Ann Woodbury, a research scientist of my staff in her DC-1 office. He asked that she destroy all copies of a memo she circulated two days previously. The memo contained a data analysis of a recent National Center for Health Statistics Survey of

Surgical Device complication rates, and the implant issues that summarized the overall scope and current status of epidemiology projects for the Health Care Business's mammary implant products.

Mary Ann asked me to join them in her office and Greg repeated his request to both of us. Greg stated to us that he was acting at the specific request of Robert Rylee II, vice-president and general manager of the health care business, who was very angry with the memos, and that he had spoken with Mr. Rylee on this subject earlier by telephone. He also stated that from his personal viewpoint, the information contained in the memos would compromise projects that he was then working on in Dow Corning product liability litigation and be adverse to the company if publicly revealed. I directed Mary Ann not [to] comply with the request and stated to Greg that to do so would in my opinion be unethical conduct.

I feel that this is a serious example of misconduct requiring formal review. I am concerned that these documents may be sought out and destroyed. Also, I am concerned that the incident, if not amended, may lead to others that would threaten the integrity of my department, its employees, their ability to provide valid scientific evaluations to management, as well as their careers in the company. I therefore ask the committee's review of this matter.

In his 14 years on the company's Business Conduct Committee, Swanson often had been asked by employees to look into a variety of personal and company-related problems. They would jot him a memo or call him on the telephone with every complaint imaginable, from charges of sexual harassment to inquiries about how the company's purchasing agents should deal with invitations from suppliers. When the company's Mexican subsidiary ran a want ad for a "sexo masculino" chemical engineer, he was asked whether discriminatory hiring was a violation of the code of conduct. It was a violation and was immediately corrected. When an employee was arrested after a barroom brawl that ended in a high-speed chase through Midland's streets, Swanson was asked to deter-

mine whether the company should set "boundaries" or guidelines for behavior outside of work. The committee decided
against such an intrusion into the private lives of its employees. But rarely had Swanson received a memo with so serious
a charge as Dillon's, and never one that was so openly
accusatory.

At Dow Corning, direct confrontations were rare. When
executives disagreed with one another, they did so politely and
with soft voices. They rarely put their disagreements on paper,
and they virtually never engaged in face-to-face conflicts. The
company's culture was genteel, full of polite smiles and informal hallway meetings—the corporate version of the Stepford
wife syndrome. At Dow Corning, compromise and consensus
weren't an art. They were *the* corporate way of life for virtually
every successful manager and executive.

For someone like Dillon to accuse a top executive of
attempting to quash information damaging to the company
was more than highly unusual. It was nearly reckless. Dillon
had worked at the company for only three years. He was generally known as an unflappable, quiet doctor and manager
who only spoke up in meetings when he had something worth
saying. Either Dillon was so outraged by the incident that he
threw all caution to the wind, or he was simply politically
naive and idealistic in taking on the powerful Rylee, who had
built a reputation as a savvy, tough, and outspoken executive
over more than a dozen years at Dow Corning.

*   *   *

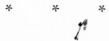

While Dillon and Rylee were opposites in personality and
background, both were anomalies within Dow Corning's culture. A native of San Francisco, Dillon had studied at
Berkeley in the late sixties and early seventies when the university became a center of unrest and protest. Indeed, his
friends must have wondered if Dillon ever wanted to leave the
university because he studied there for more than a decade.
After earning an undergraduate degree in anthropology in

1968, he stayed to get a master's in the subject, along with a master's in public health and a Ph.D. in medical anthropology. He finished his last Berkeley degree in late 1975.

Dillon seemed to drift here and there before joining Dow Corning as medical director in July 1987. He spent one year in a post-doctoral fellowship program at the University of California's San Francisco Medical School. He moved across country to teach epidemiology and research design at East Carolina University for a year before going to medical school at Chicago's Rush Medical College. His residency in internal medicine was done at Bertram Medical Center in Pittsfield, Massachusetts. He joined General Electric Company in its Pittsfield clinic in 1984, where he practiced occupational medicine until he moved to Dow Corning. As medical director, he supervised the company's epidemiological studies and oversaw its medical information systems, among other things.

Vice-president Rylee, by contrast, was a shrewd former trial attorney, a seasoned country lawyer who had outfoxed many opponents in courtrooms with a quick wit and a sharp tongue. He grew up in Dennison, a small Texas town just north of Dallas, did a two-year hitch in the army during the Korean conflict, and then went to the University of Texas law school. Rylee was handling malpractice and corporate law in Corpus Christi for a little over a decade when his stepfather, the founder and owner of Wright Manufacturing, a small company in Memphis that made stainless steel hip replacements, suffered a severe heart attack in 1967.

Rylee had helped his stepfather with a few things in the past, usually dispensing some lawyerly advice. Now, he was asked to take over the business. He began commuting back and forth between Corpus Christi and Memphis, until he decided there was an interesting future with Wright Manufacturing, which then was generating little more than $500,000 a year in sales. In mid-1968, when Dillon was still a student on one of the country's most turbulent and volatile campuses, Rylee resigned his law partnership, moved to Memphis, and became chief executive of his stepfather's company.

He spent little time looking back. Rylee enjoyed being the

man in charge, learning more about the spare body part business. In the early days, he made it a practice to spend two or three mornings a week at Baptist Hospital in Memphis where he would scrub in surgery, don a green gown and cap, and watch a doctor replace a hip with one of his company's prostheses. He became the first nonsurgeon to take a course on total hip replacements from a pioneer in the operation in England. He expanded the product line to knees. He even received four patents on four surgical instruments used in total knee replacement surgery.

By 1977, Wright Manufacturing was selling nearly $4 million worth of knee and hip replacements when Rylee decided to cash in on the business. Johnson & Johnson and 3M were interested in Wright. But it was Dow Corning that seemed to offer the greatest promise and potential for growth. Wright would have been just another tiny appendage of a J&J or 3M. At Dow Corning, however, it would become the vehicle to cultivate and market a broad range of medical products—from silicone finger joints and breast implants to Wright's own spare body parts. As an industrial chemical company, Dow Corning never really knew how to market to doctors and hospitals. Rylee and his company—with its sales force of 35 people selling directly to orthopedic surgeons and operating room supervisors—would bring that expertise.

Rylee was impressed with the integrity of Chief Executive Officer Ludington, who had initiated and championed Dow Corning's code of ethics and a set of basic values to guide the behavior of the company's executives. So Rylee sold his firm to Dow Corning in 1977 and remained as president of what was renamed Dow Corning Wright. If Si Braley was responsible for getting Dow Corning into the breast implant business, Bob Rylee was instrumental in making the company the market leader in this small plastic surgery niche. Within a year of the acquisition, Rylee was responsible for marketing, sales, and distribution of the breast implants, which were made at Dow Corning's Hemlock plant, some 20 miles from the company's Midland headquarters. He built a direct sales force to call on plastic surgeons, replacing the network of dealers and hospital supply houses Dow Corning had relied upon. Sales began to climb—even in the face of tougher competition. By 1984, the company moved some research and development people for breast implants to Memphis, and, in 1988, it began to manufacture some breast implants there. Rylee, meantime, moved up the corporate ladder to become general manager of Dow Corning's health care businesses in 1980. Seven years later, he was awarded a corporate vice-presidency, and in 1990, he was named chairman of all the company's health care products.

On December 14, 1990, Rylee was in an airplane flying home to Memphis from Midland when he opened his briefcase and pulled out the material that research scientist Mary Ann Woodbury had distributed a few hours earlier. The corporation was already under increasing pressure due to breast implants and Rylee was bearing the brunt of it. An adversarial relationship had developed between the company and the FDA regarding the issue—thanks to all the prodding by Sidney Wolfe, Command Trust Network, and other activists. Word was getting out that the FDA would soon require Dow Corning and other implant makers to prove the safety and effectiveness of breast implants or yank them off the market. Less than a month earlier, the company had lost its lawsuit with Public Citizen to keep the safety studies it had given to the FDA under wraps. The Connie Chung segment on the dangers of implants had aired just four days earlier. In another four days, Rylee was to fly to Washington to testify before a hostile House subcommittee on the safety of the devices.

Ironically, one of the reasons for Woodbury's evaluation was to help prepare Rylee for his appearance before Congress. She was supposed to present her analysis before Rylee and the other members of a recently created group, internally dubbed the Reed Committee, which was to handle what was fast becoming a crisis over breast implants. The group of high-level executives, chaired by Dow Corning Chief Executive Larry Reed, included Rylee and United States area Vice-President Kerm Campbell, the man John Swanson would later approach to request his recusal. It also included general counsel James Jenkins, Dr. Robert R. LeVier, technical director of the health care businesses, and a host of additional legal and communication staffers.

Though Reed was the highest ranking official in the group, Rylee had gradually evolved into the company's top spokesperson on breast implants. It wasn't that Rylee was all that adept at media relations, but he was the best foot the company could put forward. Reed, described by many as aloof and wooden, was not an imposing executive. Lanky and rather awkward, he had a weak voice and when he spoke about important matters, he somehow made them sound almost trivial. Rylee presented a more polished image. He was personable and quick on his feet, and he had a knack for making fairly inno-cuous statements sound important. "The reason he was the front man was because he was the best at it," says Arnold Zenker, the communications consultant who helped train Dow Corning executives. "He was more comfortable at it. He was articulate. We understood that he could look too slick, that he could look too unconcerned. But some of those other guys would have collapsed in a heap."

Dillon and Woodbury had been scheduled to make their presentation before the Reed Committee on Wednesday, December 12—two days before the incident that caused Dillon to write his complaint to Swanson. But other issues had taken up so much of the committee's afternoon that Woodbury had simply circulated her memos at the session's conclusion.

So Rylee didn't know of Woodbury's assessment—that the company was significantly underestimating the number of complaints and complications caused by breast implants—until Friday, when he was flying home to Memphis. Immediately, Rylee went ballistic. Lawyers were already crawling all over the company's files, looking for documents that would bolster their product liability cases against Dow Corning. As a former attorney, Rylee quickly realized what damage such a memo could cause in front of a jury sympathetic to a suffering woman and antagonistic to a big, faceless corporation.

Woodbury, evaluating a 1988 survey of implanted devices by the National Center for Health Statistics, reported that 30.3 percent of women with implants experienced problems with them. Roughly 13 percent of the sampled population had their implants replaced within five years, while an additional 17 percent had them replaced within 10 years. "Defect or malfunction was given as a reason for replacement in 30 percent of the replaced devices," Woodbury noted. Rylee and other Dow Corning officials were publicly saying that breast implant complication rates were far lower—that implant ruptures, for example, occurred in fewer than 1 percent of cases. It was an especially sensitive issue because some FDA officials suspected that the manufacturers were purposely overestimating the number of women with implants in order to arrive at a lower percentage rate of complications. Dillon and several of his staffers were already skeptical of the complication rates Rylee would commonly cite. "I just didn't think we knew what the true number was...," said Dillon, who thought the company should make a better effort to find out.

Rylee was just one of about a dozen people at Dow Corning who received the Woodbury memo. As soon as he could, Rylee called the legal department in Midland and asked that a lawyer visit with the epidemiologist in Dillon's medical services department, about three miles from Dow Corning's corporate center. Woodbury became, in Dillon's words, "extremely upset" when Greg Thiess, a corporate attorney assigned to breast implant litigation, showed up at her office and asked that she "withdraw" the document. Thiess was a tall, gangly workaholic who always seemed hurried and preoccupied. With a sober-looking Thiess still in her office, Woodbury rushed out to get Dillon for support. "She just said that he was making requests and that she didn't feel that she could handle it, and she wanted me to come in and join her...in the discussion."

Dillon walked across the hallway to Woodbury's office, and Thiess reiterated his demand that the memos be "retrieved and withdrawn." But when Dillon pressed him on what exactly was wrong with the documents, the lawyer was vague. He said he was acting upon Rylee's specific request and that Rylee was very angry about the memo's contents. Dillon offered to write a correcting memo if Thiess believed that Woodbury's analysis was inaccurate or misrepresented the complication data.

Thiess, however, simply said the memos were inappropriate. He said Rylee agreed and so did Donald R. Weyenberg, the company's vice-president of research and development, whom Thiess had bumped into that afternoon in the hall.

"Look," Dillon said finally, "I think this is an ethical problem. It's improper to just drop into somebody's office and ask to recall memos."

Dillon then asked the lawyer to leave. Both he and Woodbury were incredulous that a vice-president of the company would want an internal memo designed to help the firm destroyed. "We were all very concerned about it," said Dillon. "It was very upsetting.... It was a kind of unprecedented thing. I never really heard of anything like this happening before.... It seemed to me that this was just a very basic issue. It just seemed like a very necessary piece of information we needed for scientific purposes. If something as simple as this could be so controversial, I didn't really see how we could even get any studies done.... I don't think under any circumstances ever would I have let these memos be destroyed."

Just four days later, on December 18, Rylee sat before a House subcommittee. "Dow Corning," he testified, "has not and would not keep important evidence of a health risk from FDA and surgeons who have the professional responsibility to discuss all risk with their patients...our ethics, and our code of business conduct as employees of this corporation, would demand that we report evidence of a health risk, should one ever be discovered from our research."

On December 20, Dillon was still so angry about the incident in Woodbury's office that he wrote and sent his memo to Swanson requesting a formal investigation by the company's Business Conduct Committee.

*   *   *

As Swanson sat at his own desk, reading the complaint on Dow Corning stationery from Dillon, he was astounded by the charge. At home, he was still debating with Colleen the pros and cons of having her implants taken out. She was getting increasingly bitter toward the company as they both began to wonder if Dow Corning had known of the risks and hazards and failed to properly inform patients of them. Dillon's memo was a small piece of the puzzle that made Swanson more curious and suspicious about what was going on.

The memo provided few details of exactly what transpired or even what kind of complication rates on breast implants were being reported by Woodbury. So Swanson was as intrigued by what wasn't in the memo as he was by its contents. After the holidays, the Business Conduct Committee set up a January 3 meeting to discuss the incident. Swanson, eager to find out more about what had happened, called Woodbury that morning on the telephone.

"I want to let you know we have a meeting set up for this afternoon and I'm hoping we will have our whole committee," he told Woodbury. "One of the questions that will come up is what is the nature of the information that is in question here. Can you give me just a brush-stroke idea of what it is we're talking about that Bob Rylee is so concerned about?"

Woodbury explained that she had studied the complaint data from Dow Corning Wright's own files as well as from other sources, including the government. In her analysis, she had noted that complaints received by the company probably represented only a portion of the actual number because "it's only those that get back to us through a doctor's office." Some surgeons don't report all problems or complaints, and there was no requirement to do so. Woodbury also believed that the company overestimated the number of people with breast implants, which would automatically lower the percentage with reported problems. "Its net effect is probably a substantial underassessment of the actual complaint rate," she told Swanson.

"So you were looking at it in kind of an outside-in or more objective way, questioning whether the use of that data was accurate and representative?" asked Swanson. "And Bob took issue with that?"

"Apparently. The other one was a memo that is an analysis of data that is publicly available. We purchased a computer tape from the National Center for Health Statistics on a sample of people who received a medical device of some sort and they were then asked a series of questions about complications and replacements. We knew there was going to be a publicly issued report coming out with at least a portion of that data. We had done an assessment of that tape to provide Rylee with preliminary information so he would know what to expect."

"But this was publicly available data. Why would anyone in our company have a problem with that?" asked Swanson. "Sidney Wolfe could get hold of that as easily as we could, I assume."

"Yes," answered Woodbury, "anybody can get it and analyze the data. We did the actual analysis."

"It was our interpretation of it that was in question?"

"I did not provide any interpretation. I provided only analysis and what I felt were the limitations of the data but I drew no conclusions whatsoever."

"And that was a problem for Bob, too?"

"He wanted that withdrawn as well," replied Woodbury.

"Even from presentation to our own people, our biosafety committee?"

"Yes."

"Did he give you any reason for this?" asked Swanson.

"We never spoke directly," she replied. "This was through Greg. His concern was...that there were internal memos that were being used in court against us. He said those can end up being called into court and into the FDA and so forth and statements that we made about the product and complication rates could cause some problems in court. I can understand his concerns from a legal standpoint, but that doesn't make it not true."

"I think we have an obligation here to look at our own information and our own assessment of it with some objectivity," Swanson told her. "We're not talking about making it public here, but making it available to the management of the company, the people who have to make decisions here, and that's probably the basis of your concern."

"Yes, it is, definitely," she said.

The issue wasn't resolved that afternoon. Instead, another meeting was scheduled for January 9 at which everyone involved in the incident would give their views. Although Swanson created the session's agenda, he was asked by Richard A. Hazleton, then general manager of the company's industrial products group, if he would mind not attending the meeting. Though taken aback, Swanson didn't put up a fight—perhaps because he knew he was beginning to be conflicted on the issue due to Colleen's worsening condition. "I felt hurt," he recalls. "I was surprised, but I tried to play it cool. I didn't ask why, and I know I should have. It was a mistake. I should have confronted him right then and there, but I think Dick knew by then that I was empathetic to Dillon's position. I liked Chuck and at least on the basis of his memo felt that he had raised a legitimate ethical issue. I tended to be very supportive of his concerns, and I think that was understood."

At the meeting, it became clear that attorney Thiess, who had demanded the destruction of Woodbury's analysis, was simply following Rylee's orders, and most of the time was spent going over exactly what had happened. The memo detailing the session—as is customary at most corporations—took all the emotion and all the blood out of the confrontation. Summing up the meeting, Hazleton and Jere Marciniak, another member of the conduct committee, wrote: "Bob Rylee indicated that when he received the information in question on the way back to Memphis, he was very concerned that the way it was stated was prejudicial to Dow Corning's interests and could have adverse impact in future litigation situations. He stated he did not intend in this case, nor does he advocate in general, suppressing either factual information or professional conclusions or opinions. He does believe it is important to have documentation that, in its complete form, makes as clear as possible the distinctions between facts, conclusions or opinions of people inside and outside Dow Corning with which Dow Corning agrees, and conclusions or opinions which Dow Corning does not agree."

Another outcome of the meeting was that the incident would be used as a springboard for the development of a set of guidelines about how disagreements about the content of corporate documents should be addressed in the future. "To resolve the specifics of these events," wrote Hazleton and Marciniak, "Mary Ann Woodbury agreed to forward another copy of the documents in question to Bob Rylee. He in turn will document his concerns relating to possible misinterpretation of the information in the documents and the possible damage to Dow Corning which could ensue."

Swanson was bitterly disappointed in the meeting's outcome. He believed that his Business Conduct Committee colleagues had skirted the real issue of whether the company was deliberately underestimating the complication rates for a controversial product by focusing instead on a corporate policy for how disagreements should be handled in the future. "There were two broad issues," Swanson says. "First, the process and protocol for how people deal with sensitive information they don't particularly like. But second, there was the content issue. What was it about the survey information itself that was so scary to Rylee? The content issue was essentially ignored."

Indeed, even though Swanson was sent the original complaint, he had a difficult time getting hold of the record of the meeting. He had to write several memos himself before receiving a copy of the new policy on documents.

Dillon wasn't happy, either. Although he believed the meeting cleared up some misunderstandings, he left the session skeptical that research studies he had been trying to get Dow Corning to do on silicone breast implants would ever be launched. Dillon and his staff had been urging Rylee to fund a variety of studies that would explore basic cancer and mortality issues, post-surgical complication rates, and whether silicone could cause immune diseases. He was going to make the argument for such studies again at the December 12 meeting that had been cut short. "The studies had been on the table for a fair amount of time, and there hadn't really been any action taken on them," he said. Some delay was caused when one of the plastic surgeons' trade groups declined to co-sponsor the research, and other implant makers also weren't eager to fund it, either. Now Dillon believed Dow Corning wouldn't go it alone. "The studies were simply not being funded or I didn't feel that they were going to be. Unlike many people at Dow Corning, I certainly had contacts with scientists and many contractors that we dealt with, and I felt very embarrassed that I'd sort of put myself out…. I spent a lot of effort in trying to get the studies funded and time was going by and nothing was happening."

Just a few months later, in April, Dillon quit his job and moved to the Boston area to set up a private medical practice. He had had it with corporate life, bureaucracy, and politics. His wife disliked living in Midland. He was frustrated by his inability to get Dow Corning to move ahead on research he thought was valuable and necessary. And he considered the Rylee incident "a jolt that just made my wife and I reassess really what we were trying to do."

A couple of weeks before Dillon's departure, Swanson had the opportunity to chat with him about silicone implants. No one inside or outside Dow Corning knew about Colleen's problems or her increasing antagonism toward the company. No one had any idea of the personal anguish that Swanson was now feeling. So Dillon answered Swanson's questions not knowing how truly interested he was in the answers.

Dillon told Swanson that he really couldn't say with certainty if silicone posed a risk to women with breast implants because the science wasn't yet complete on it. But there already was information, he said, that pointed to some problems down the road. He surmised that there probably were some women who could not tolerate silicone. Yet there was no screen to identify them in advance.

"Good luck," Dillon told Swanson when he said his good-byes. "Dow Corning is going to need a person like you."

Swanson thought it a compliment, but wondered just what he could do, and how long he could hold on.

TAKING THEM OUT

It got to be a topic at dinner every night—at least when Colleen was able to come to dinner, which was becoming less of a common occurrence. The topic was unavoidable. As the stakes grew higher for both Colleen and Dow Corning, John Swanson found it impossible to put the controversy out of his mind. During the day, at work, people around John were busy doing damage control as one implant story after another found its way into a newspaper or yet another television show. Swanson would hear his colleagues decry the idiotic bureaucrats at the FDA, the outright crazies of the Command Trust, and a sensationalistic media interested in little more than selling papers or increasing audience share. What hurt, though, were the negative, sometimes cruel, comments by fellow employees who so readily dismissed the complaints of women with implants.

In the evening, at home, Colleen was slipping closer to what seemed like slow death. Her breasts had become increasingly hard and painful. Nearly unbearable pain convulsed her left arm, hand, and ring and index fingers. Her fatigue grew worse and her interest in sex decreased. By March 1991, the pain moved into her hips and the mobility of both the right and left sides of her body declined. The ache spread to her neck and became so intense she could barely hold up her head. At home, over dinner and in bed, Swanson would hear his wife complain of a litany of health problems she believed were caused by the Dow Corning implants in her chest. And he would hear Colleen's accusations—informed in part by Anneken and the Command Trust—that his employer knew far more than it told him about the risks and dangers of implants.

She gradually came to believe that Dow Corning had been less than up-front about the risks of having implants and had denied her the right of informed consent. "I should have had a choice," she insisted. "All of the existing information about the potential risks of implants should have been available because I should have had the right to make an informed choice. If there had been one chance in a million of something going wrong, I definitely would not have had the implants. Coming from John and Si, I thought what could possibly go wrong? I believed, I trusted, and I was betrayed."

After listening with much sympathy to Colleen's concerns, Swanson would turn around and go back to work the next day—only to hear yet again the other side—that Dow Corning was an innocent victim of overzealous regulators and consumer groups. Though he had no daily role in the implant business, it seemed to find its way to his desk. In early 1991, he was asked to help draft a statement for internal use to explain why Dow Corning was staying in the breast implant business. Rylee ended up writing his own version of the statement, which included his assertion that "the reported incidence of serious complications is very small as a percentage." Commenting on the terms used by Rylee, Swanson scribbled to Robert Grupp, a colleague in the communications department: "This is *our* judgment. What is *serious?*" As the public perception took hold that Dow Corning was blocking the release of adverse health and safety information on implants, Swanson urged General Counsel James R. Jenkins to be more open and candid in the company's communications with key constituencies.

In March, when Grupp was drafting a press release to "welcome" release of the FDA's orders to companies to prove the safety and efficacy of implants, Swanson questioned Rylee's contributions again. He thought Rylee's expressed confidence that Dow Corning could satisfy the FDA that its implants were safe was unrealistic. If "the FDA still decides later this year to ban silicone implants," wrote Swanson in a memo to Grupp, "we could lose some degree of credibility. Is there a way our message—externally and internally—can consider this possibility and yet keep a positive approach?...I think Rylee's statements are overoptimistic."

Every article that came out, every bit of information he could find, he devoured. When Colleen went to bed early, Swanson would end up in his den until the wee hours of the morning. Sometimes, he would just sit there wondering how he and his wife were ever going to get through this. Most times, he would sit and read every piece of information he had gathered on silicone implants, from the latest story in the *Midland Daily News* to what few files he had on implants in his own cabinets at work. Swanson found, for example, the corporate defense he had helped draft in response to the negative *Ms.* articles published years earlier in 1977, the questions on implants he had written for the media seminar in 1978, and an internal response to a 1983 *Washington Post* story critical of implants. He began to compile a chronology of events in the breast implant crisis, often scribbling his own comments in the margins. As his doubts about the company's role increased, his written comments became more strident and severe. When the *Midland Daily News* quoted Rylee as saying the company couldn't provide more information to women with implants because, "We don't know who the patients are," Swanson sarcastically jotted in red ink: "And we don't care."

On June 1, 1991, Swanson picked up *Business Week* magazine and turned the pages to a story that would finally push him over the edge. Under the headline "Breast Implants: What Did the Industry Know, and When?," the article by journalist Tim Smart lent credence to everything Colleen had been saying about Dow Corning. It charged that the company had been aware for at least a decade of animal studies linking implants to cancer and other illnesses. The story quoted Thomas D. Talcott, a former materials engineer who claimed to have quit his job at Dow Corning in a dispute over implant safety, saying: "The manufacturers and surgeons have been performing experimental surgery on humans." Representative Ted Weiss, who held the congressional hearings on implants six months earlier, was heavily critical of the FDA for dragging its feet. "FDA documents indicate that for more than 10 years, FDA scientists expressed concerns about the safety of silicone breast implants that were frequently ignored by FDA officials," said Weiss.

The story, which appeared a few weeks before a major court battle was to begin in San Francisco between Dow Corning and a woman with implants, also detailed what it called the company's full-court press to keep internal memos and studies that surfaced in earlier court cases from reaching the public. "We don't want to be overeducating plaintiffs' attorneys," explained Bob Rylee to the reporter. It hardly seemed like the behavior of an ethical company.

Some of the information in the story would probably have been classified as proprietary or restricted inside Dow Corning. "The article put me over the edge," remembers Swanson. "It was the first time the company's ethics were questioned in a public way. To me, it was devastating. There were allegations and charges that we didn't have answers for."

Alarmed, Swanson sought to use his position as the sole permanent member of its Business Conduct Committee to change the company's hardline position. "Even though I was convinced that Colleen was affected by her implants, I was not totally convinced the corporation's position on this was altogether wrong," recalls Swanson. "I was in a position of having worked with three chief executives and having access to almost anything I wanted. I should have known where the skeletons were. That's why someone in my position sitting there reading this stuff in *Business Week* about our hidden records and what we knew for decades was just a mind-buster. It tipped the scales for me."

Swanson read the article again and again—at least three times that afternoon at his desk—before writing an e-mail note to George Callaghan, the corporate comptroller, who was then serving as the chairman of the Business Conduct Committee. "The time may have come for influence leaders in this company to come to grips with the total issue and re-examine our position," he wrote. "When a respected business publication that is well read by much of our customer base takes the stand that it has, isn't it time that we begin to look a little harder at our own position? Some 20 years ago, Dow

Chemical's intransigence about napalm gave that company a public image that took hundreds of millions of dollars and a total change in attitude to reverse. It's a lesson worth studying."

Rather than transmit the message immediately, Swanson decided to wait a day or two. Whenever he wrote an electronic message on something he felt strongly about, he had made it a habit to wait at least 24 hours before sending it. He had seen too many situations where other managers, angry over an issue, would tap out a response that would only create a hail storm of e-mail messages. Swanson wanted his memo to be meaningful and not full of emotion, a document that he wouldn't mind being read by others, from the chairman on down. With a few changes, the memo was sent on June 4 to Callaghan, and then Swanson went personally to see and speak with the two other members of the Business Conduct Committee.

Almost overnight, Swanson found himself in complete disagreement with his company. Dow Corning maintained that more than 300 studies on silicone breast implants proved the safety of the devices. However, the vast majority of these studies were not on implants, but instead on various silicone compounds, and very few, if any, of the studies examined the possibility that silicone could cause auto-immune disease. The company argued that it had provided "an ongoing flow of information" to plastic surgeons since it entered the marketplace in the early 1960s. The company said it continued to inform Washington regulators of the status and results of all its ongoing research. Responding to the *Business Week* article in a letter to the magazine's editor, United States area Vice-President Kerm Campbell wrote that the story "only serves to continue the public confusion" over implants. "*Business Week*'s responsibility for objective reporting was also compromised by the total omission of any commentary from the medical community," Campbell said.

Swanson, however, didn't buy into the company's standard responses to critics. Convinced something was terribly amiss, he began to argue in favor of suspending the sale and production of all implants until Dow Corning had time to look into the charges and thoroughly answer them. He spoke with the other members of the Business Conduct Committee and other managers at Dow Corning as well. He considered going directly to Larry Reed, the company's embattled chief executive, but decided against it after hearing that Reed was considering suing the FDA to prevent the release of company studies. Swanson also knew that Reed did not easily tolerate criticism of the company from outside sources. He was distrustful of the media and would, in Swanson's opinion, not be willing to make any substantial concessions based on the *Business Week* disclosures. In any case, Reed had delegated responsibility for managing the implant crisis to Campbell, who in effect was becoming Dow Corning's implant czar.

So Swanson instead went to see Campbell to press his position that the company should pull out of the market, at least temporarily. Not surprisingly, none of Swanson's Business Conduct colleagues agreed with him. They recognized that the company needed to look at the issue carefully, but would not commit themselves to the view that it should get out of the business. The committee members saw it as a business issue rather than an ethical issue. It didn't make economic sense for Dow Corning to withdraw a product that virtually everyone in the company believed was safe and effective. Swanson, however, believed that the company's position and actions were not only ethically off-center, but misguided even in terms of sound long-term business strategy. Unless the company toned down its strident, defensive position and at least acknowledged that there might be some women with legitimate silicone-related problems, Dow Corning would very probably become known as an insensitive corporate pariah.

To Swanson, the real issue by this time was not the accuracy of the scientific studies disclosed by *Business Week*. There was, of course, the growing belief among researchers and doctors that silicone could cause health problems. But Swanson's primary concern was that the company may not have been totally open about what it knew. "Perception, as they say, is reality," says Swanson. "And that perception was hurting the company."

Campbell, however, was far more receptive to Swanson's reasoning than most of Dow Corning's senior management. Campbell agreed that immediately suspending of the breast implant business was probably the right thing to do under the circumstances, Swanson recalls, but he was uneasy about the legal implications. If Dow Corning halted sales and production, would it only serve to undermine the company's position in court? General Counsel Jenkins and his legal staff already had become hardliners on the issue, according to a former top executive. They insisted that the company should hold firm and refuse to publicly release the company's safety studies on the grounds that disclosure would damage its competitive position. And Jenkins—along with most of Dow Corning's senior executives—certainly would not have favored the idea of halting the manufacture and sale of implants at that time.

A board of directors' meeting was scheduled in Midland for June 10, 1991. It was well understood that the directors would come to the meeting with hard questions about the charges leveled against Dow Corning in the *Business Week* article. Swanson recommended to Campbell that a pre-emptive statement be prepared for the board to consider. Campbell agreed and on June 6—just two days after his e-mail message to colleagues—Swanson wrote a proposed news release under the headline: "Dow Corning Wright to Suspend Production of Mammary Implants."

> Dow Corning announced that its subsidiary company, Dow Corning Wright, will temporarily suspend the production and sale of silicone mammary implants until research on certain issues has been concluded. Since entering the market in 1963, Dow Corning has continuously studied the health and safety effects of these devices. "We believe our breast implants are safe and pose no significant health risk," said J. Kermit Campbell, Dow Corning group vice-president, USA. "But we recognize that questions about the safety of silicone implants exist and we are placing a high priority on finding scientifically sound answers to these questions."

By now, Swanson didn't believe the silicone implants were safe. But if he had written anything more negative, he believed, there would not have been a chance to even get a hearing. Campbell apparently took Swanson's press release to the board meeting on June 10, but did not vigorously lobby in favor of its position, according to sources. The meeting lasted more than four hours. Ultimately, the board was swayed by the attorneys' arguments that to suspend operations could be interpreted as an admission of a product problem and could potentially damage the company in the courts. Besides, the company was still confident that the tens of thousands of pages of research studies and other information it was preparing to provide to the FDA a month later, on July 8, would satisfy the agency that implants were safe and effective.

Disheartened by the decision, Swanson wondered what he had spent his life promoting. As the company's guardian of ethics, he had helped to build a tremendous amount of good will among its employees. His own department's employee attitude surveys showed that in 1988 more than 90 percent of Dow Corning's United States employees believed the company to be a highly-ethical corporation. But more than a violation of ethics, he viewed the board's decision as a colossal blunder. "I was angry at the shortsightedness of the company and the lack of leadership and vision at the top," he recalls. "I thought it was the worst decision the company could have made and that the corporation would never again be the same. I was convinced that at some point or another, the company would be materially affected. It had already forfeited much of its reputation in the public eye. I felt it was the beginning of a long, slow process of financial deterioration. My trust level in the company was rapidly eroding."

He had no ethical qualms about playing an active role in the crisis, even as his wife was accusing the company of fraud in their private conversations. Swanson never bought into the notion that employees should serve their companies with blind loyalty. "I never believed that, and I never will," he says. "I suppose there was some personal conflict for me, but I felt that I could deal with it and live with it." Indeed, he believed that there were times when employees could best serve their organizations by acting in ways that some might consider disloyal. He always encouraged employees not to fear making unpopular choices if they believed something was amiss and had reasonable cause for their concerns. In fact, he considered it an employee's moral imperative to speak up against a perceived wrong. "Corporate political correctness says that once you reach a consensus in a group, everyone should support the group view," says Swanson. "But listening to the minority opinion is extraordinarily valuable in many cases, even when it borders on allegations of disloyalty. I was trying to be constructive in my time left with the company by being, in a sense, disloyal—disloyal only because I disagreed with our management. I had what I thought were sound reasons to disagree, and they were not exclusively related to Colleen's problems. They had to do with the ethical rightness of how Dow Corning was deciding to manage its way through this issue."

Swanson's philosophy about the meaning of loyalty is one not commonly found in management or career books. He was aware that his was, at best, a contrarian view. "Speaking out about sensitive company issues is not a career-building modus operandi," he says. "But it was the only way I could live with myself."

Though Swanson still told no one of his wife's problems, he became less hesitant about sharing his position on implants with others at the company, including Dan Hayes, a close friend who was then president and chief executive of Dow Corning Wright. Hayes, in Midland for the board meeting, also was upset with the directors, but for an entirely different reason. Though the board spent hours discussing breast implants, Hayes was present only for a short period of time—even though he was the top executive of the subsidiary that made and sold the devices. He had been asked to leave the session because he was not a director.

When Swanson and Hayes agreed to meet at the Midland Country Club for a late-afternoon nine holes of golf, breast implants dominated their conversation. They had been friends for two decades. They shared not only an employer, but also a passion for the game of golf that over the years had brought them together in numerous club-sponsored tournaments and matches.

On occasion Swanson would represent the corporate Business Conduct Committee and visit Memphis to talk to Dow Corning Wright employees about the company's ethics program. Hayes, of course, would attend and participate in these meetings. "In retrospect," says Swanson, "I probably should have taken myself out of some of these because I was too close to Dan. I think I was probably too sympathetic to the issues he was facing." None of the audits, however, had ever turned up any evidence of serious problems with breast implants.

Swanson recalls an unusual request from Dow Corning's executive committee in late 1986 to audit how Dow Corning Wright planned, conducted, and controlled clinical trials for new products. He had not been involved in the investigation, which was performed by two other members of the Business Conduct Committee. Nor did he receive the results of the audit, although a former executive says the review was done only to find out why new medical products were often on a speedier schedule for approval and release than the company's industrial products. The reason: Compe-tition was far more severe in the medical device industry. Still, Swanson wondered if his friendship with Hayes had somehow compromised other audits of Dow Corning Wright in which he was involved.

Hayes already had an indication of how Swanson felt about the issue of breast implants. A few days before the board meeting on June 10, Hayes and Robert R. LeVier, technical director of the health care businesses, were speaking to Dow Corning staffers at an employee forum at corporate headquarters. To support his position that implants were safe, Hayes quoted a recent study sponsored by the American Society of Plastic and Reconstructive Surgeons that Swanson knew was flawed. Swanson had come across the study—of 100,000 house-holds—months earlier, when Dow Corning used it as a "back-grounder" for the media. It showed that 92.5 percent of the respondents said they were satisfied with the results of their implant surgery, and 82 percent said that without a doubt, they would choose to have the surgery once again. Nowhere did Dow Corning report that the survey was based on only 441 responses, or a response rate of under 0.5 percent, which made its results highly suspect and statistically invalid.

After the presentation, Swanson told Hayes he believed the statistics from the plastic surgeons' group were misleading, in any case, because they were based on such a small response rate.

On the golf course, after the board meeting, the two friends thoroughly debated the issue. "We spent a few hours playing golf, talking, arguing, discussing this whole thing," says Swanson. Hayes took the position, that there was no need for Dow Corning to get out of the business. To temporarily halt the sale and manufacture of implants would immediately kill the entire business, Hayes argued. "After that discussion, it was clear there was no room for agreement between Dan and me," says Swanson. "We agreed to disagree."

Swanson was beginning to feel a little like a lone salmon swimming upstream.

*   *   *

At the time, Hayes was in the midst of the storm, desperately trying to orchestrate a grass-roots campaign that would bring together other implant makers, the plastic surgeons, and women satisfied with their implants to offset the mounting criticism. In a memo to his colleagues two weeks after the board meeting, Hayes apparently felt the company was succeeding in keeping the lid on more damaging coverage in the media. "The issue of cover-up is going well from a long-term perspective," he wrote in the memo dated June 24, 1991.

Still, Swanson's friend was clearly worried that Dow Corning was far behind in establishing these networks of contacts to support its position. "The number one issue in my mind is the establishment of networks," he added. "I believe we have made no progress in the two weeks. Obviously, this is the largest single issue on our platter because it affects not only the next 2–3 years profitability of DCC (Dow Corning Corporation), but also ultimately has a big impact on the long-term ethics and believability issues.... It has become obvious to me that what is at risk here is somewhere between $50 million and $500 million. Right now, I think we are losing the time race badly in this critical area, and I believe that the amount of money we are going to lose is increasing rapidly since we are not going to be in a position to divert the opposing forces into the directions we want soon."

What Hayes did not know was that Colleen Swanson could well be considered one of those "opposing forces." Swanson didn't tell Hayes that Colleen would soon have her own implants removed. Kathleen Anneken, co-founder of the Command Trust Network, had recommended that Colleen contact Lu-Jean Feng, head of microvascular surgery at Mount Sinai Medical Center in Cleveland. Feng, a diminutive, Chinese-born plastic surgeon, was one of fewer than a handful of doctors known to Anneken at the time who would remove implants without insisting that they be replaced. A clinical assistant professor of surgery at Case Western University, Feng was removing breast implants from the chests of hundreds of women every year—a practice that caused her to be vilified by many of her colleagues.

But the soft-spoken Feng, then in her late 30s, was something of a maverick. She had come to the United States with her then 45-year-old father, who had piloted a bomber for the Chinese Air Force during World War II. Feng's father viewed education as his route to stability. He earned a degree in accounting and used it to develop a new career and life for himself in the United States. He inculcated in his only child, who was in the eighth grade when they arrived in the United States, the notion that she had to rely on her instincts and her smarts.

Feng went to Yale University at the age of 16, graduating cum laude in 1975 with a bachelor's degree in molecular biophysics and biochemistry. She earned her medical degree from Yale's School of Medicine in 1979 at the age of 24. While she was at Yale, she met a female surgeon who quickly became her role model. Feng discovered that she enjoyed the craft of surgery. "I found that I liked things that are difficult," she says. "In surgery, you can make something and have a big impact on someone's life. You can also fail to improve a person. I find the risk-taking exciting."

While James Baker, who had performed the implant surgery on Colleen, was lured to plastic surgery by his own accident and his childhood interest in art, Feng was drawn into the profession by her emotions and her instincts. She enjoyed vascular and heart surgery so much she once thought she wanted to do heart transplants. "But I found that the stress becomes so much greater when you're working with very sick patients," she says. "A lot of unpredictable things can happen. Plastic surgery is more predictable. You are generally operating on healthy people to make them better. It's very artistic, and you can see the improvement you're making."

After a three-year residency in surgery at the University of California Hospital in San Francisco, Feng moved back across the country and completed a residency in plastic surgery at North Carolina Memorial Hospital in Chapel Hill. She followed that experience with a two-year fellowship at New York University with William Shaw, a superb and unconventional surgeon who pioneered the use of a person's own body tissue to rebuild the breast. She was keenly interested in microvascular surgery—largely because it was far more technically demanding and intricate work. At the time, Shaw, who was also Chinese-born, was doing microvascular surgery in the cosmetic arena. He and Feng had met at a plastic surgeons' meeting where she presented a paper on white blood cell infections. She impressed him as a "very intelligent and very serious" surgeon and soon after accepted her as a fellow. At New York University, they performed some highly complicated work together, from reattaching severed limbs to reconstructing a patient's esophagus using tissue from the bowel. "She was very skillful as a surgeon," Shaw recalls, "and she is an intense person who puts 100 percent into everything she does."

During the fellowship, both Feng and Shaw began to notice that a lot of patients came to him complaining of problems with silicone implants. Rather than replace the implants with another set, Shaw, in the early 1980s, became one of the first United States surgeons to use tissue from a woman's buttocks or abdomen to reconstruct her breasts. He became one of the first plastic surgeons known to Command Trust's Anneken who would remove a woman's implants without insisting that they be replaced by another set. Indeed, his willingness to do so, believes Shaw, who is now at UCLA, caused the California Society of Plastic Surgeons to reject his membership in 1992, even though he had been in practice as a surgeon for 15 years and had been chairman of UCLA's plastic surgery department for three years. "There were vicious rumors going around that I was charging high fees and taking out implants from patients who didn't need them taken out," says Shaw. "It wasn't true and no one ever called me directly about it. But then the society denied my membership."

Before he began removing them, Shaw had put breast implants into the chests of as many as 200 patients over the years. "If I knew it was a bad thing, I wouldn't have done one," he says. "But I also began to see the complications of implants directly because I was getting some of the most difficult cases." Taking them out was no big issue to him. "We didn't put implants in to save a patient's life. It's not like a heart valve. We put them in to make a patient happier. So the patient should have the option to have them out. Most plastic surgeons then felt falsely guilty to be involved in removing implants. They felt that because they put them in, taking them out was a defeat. I saw some of the complications of implant surgeries and realized that ultimately the patient has to decide for herself."

When Anneken asked him to recommend a few more surgeons to whom Command Trust could refer others, Shaw immediately suggested Feng, by then working as a plastic surgeon at Mount Sinai Medical Center in Cleveland and Roger Khouri in St. Louis. Feng, who had put silicone implants into about 30 patients since first practicing plastic surgery in 1987, met Anneken and Goldrich in Baltimore, Maryland, at an FDA medical device conference in February 1991. She listened to several critics of silicone breast implants discuss the possibility of silicone-immune toxicity and auto-immune illnesses and realized that far more women than she thought were having problems with the devices. "That's when I realized that there were a lot of unknowns about the implants," she says. "The can of worms opened up for me there, and right after that I started seeing my first patients."

Her decision did not surprise her old mentor. "She was objective and willing to listen to patients," says Shaw. "She wasn't going to accept the party line. And she was well trained in microsurgery and breast reconstruction so that she was ready to offer some solutions for patients who had problems with implants. She could transplant tissue from the buttocks and abdomen as needed."

A month after the conference, Feng performed her first explant on a young woman in her twenties from Montana. The patient had gotten polyurethane-coated implants five years earlier and wanted them out. She suffered several classic symptoms, including joint pain, fatigue, and memory loss, but also had broken out severely in acne and hives. "She said the minute the implants went in she felt a change in her body," says Feng. Rather than simply remove the implants, Feng decided, at the suggestion of Pierre Blais, a Canadian scientist and outspoken critic of implants, that she also should cut out all the scar tissue that had formed around the devices. Blais has examined hundreds of removed implants and claims that the devices were often manufactured under poor quality controls. Because the polyurethane foam surrounding the implant can degrade into scar tissue, Blais suggested that Feng take out all the scar tissue.

Feng found her first operation remarkably easy. "There were no guidelines on how you should take out a polyurethane implant," she says. "Technically, it was not a demanding operation. Yet, the patient got an excellent result in terms of symptoms relief. It was a defining moment for me." Further study of removed scar tissue by her colleagues found that often there were silicone crystals embedded in the human tissue.

"So you figure if it's potentially causing problems, then you have to do a more complete removal even though it's more work. If I was going to stick my neck out, I thought I should do it painstakingly right."

Because Feng did few silicone implants, she had no emotional or financial involvement in them. "I was basically a trauma surgeon who did a lot of microvascular work," she says. "When I did breast surgery, I usually put in their own tissue. I think that's what made it easier for me to explant."

Almost immediately, however, Feng found herself on the opposite side of a growing controversy from most of her plastic surgeon colleagues. Most surgeons, however, oppose explantations because they do not believe that silicone implants cause systemic illness. Why then, they argue, should you remove an implant, only to worsen a patient's appearance? "Being a woman really helped me," believes Feng. "I could understand their concerns and feelings. There are patients who you know wouldn't tell a lie and can document illnesses that developed after implantation. These illnesses became very similar from case to case, and they weren't just made up.

"I have never said there is a scientific cause and effect," Feng says. "What I say to patients is that we don't know how silicone causes this problem. We don't know if it does, but the possibility exists that it can. After a while we were just inundated with patients who wanted to find a doctor who would listen to them and not tell them they were crazy. Women were getting a pat on the head and being told, 'Honey you're really okay. Why don't you do some aerobic exercises and it will go away?'"

At Mount Sinai, Feng quickly ran into resistance. She says the hospital's chief of plastic surgery, Dr. Bahman Guyuron, argued that an explantation was an experimental procedure requiring the approval of a special committee concerned with ethics. Feng surmounted the hurdle by showing him that even Dow Corning recommended the removal of implants if a patient is suffering from immune-response symptoms such as joint pain, myositis, fever, weight loss, and other problems. Later, she says, Guyuron of plastic surgery tried to quash a paper she and others authored on the pathology of scar tissue Feng removed from patients. Some of her patients' medical records and hospital charts were reexamined by the chief's staff, she believes, in efforts to discredit her. In front of the hospital's chief executive, the chief accused her of making up patient histories in support of her report, Feng says. "It was like the cultural revolution where they just wanted to create the perception that I was dishonest by claiming I falsified patient histories and operating reports. People were suddenly looking at me with a magnifying glass to see what mistakes, if any, I might make."

Guyuron concedes that he began to investigate Feng's records for the study only after an employee on her staff came to him and suggested the research was flawed. "I found that the study was not designed properly and that some of the statements in it were unfounded," he maintains. "The study was revised and altered to a level I was comfortable with." Guyuron, who left Mount Sinai in late 1993, says he never objected to Feng's explant operations. Instead, he opposed Feng's decision to remove scar tissue from women whose breast implants had already been taken out. "There is no scientific value to that surgery," argues Guyuron. "We don't have any clear clues whether there is any relationship between implants and systemic diseases." Feng says she performed a few of these operations to remove any silicone that had been left in the body after an explantation. In 1992, before she was to attend a meeting of the Ohio Valley Plastic Surgeons Society, Feng received a telephone call from her old mentor, Shaw, who warned her that she might be attacked and accused of charging exorbitant fees for explantations. That issue and others surfaced after an Associated Press story noted that there was a Cleveland surgeon—not identified by name—who was an expert at explantation operations. Feng typically charges what medical insurance will pay for the operation—between $8000 and $10,000, based on its difficulty. She flew to the conference in Pittsburgh and faced a barrage of inquiries about her practice and her fees. She found herself on the receiving end of a series of stinging inquiries from Dr. Norman Cole, then president of the American Society of Plastic and Reconstructive Surgeons. According to Feng, he publicly lectured and reprimanded her in front of hundreds of plastic surgeons. "How can you call your- self a breast implant removal expert?," Cole asked. "You mean we can't do this? We have to go to special training to do this?"

Intimidated by the ferocity of the attacks on her integrity, Feng sought the counsel of an attorney, who advised her to document everything she did. At times, she seriously reconsid- ered what she was doing. "But what really gave me all the encouragement were my patients. They were the source of my inspiration. My patients have been provosts at universities, judges, lawyers, doctors. They are people who have a lot of integrity. This is an operation for them. When you can see patients getting better from this operation, how bad could it be?" Feng, who says more than 60 percent of her patients show improvement after an explantation, also received consid- erable support from her father. "When I met a tremendous amount of resistance over silicone, he said, 'You have to expect that people are going to fight you and you have to just hang in there. Follow your instincts. Do what you believe is right.'"

*   *   *

But all that still lay ahead when Feng received a telephone call from Colleen Swanson in April 1991. Colleen spent nearly an hour on the phone with Feng, providing every detail of her medical condition, from the early migraines and numbness in the limbs to her frozen shoulder and joint pains, from her loss of appetite and her diminished sex drive to her body rashes and chronic fatigue. Even before examining her, Feng suggest- ed that they schedule the explantation. If a full examination proved removal wasn't necessary or Colleen changed her mind for any reason, they could cancel the surgery at the last minute. It was scheduled for June 28, 1991.

The Swansons didn't want anyone at Dow Corning—or for that matter, anyone at all—to know why they were planning to travel to Cleveland. By then, Colleen had quit her job selling residential real estate and had begun caring for three infants in her home. It was far less strenuous than selling real estate, and the mothers would bring their children directly to the Swansons' home. But sometimes she would feel so weak that she could barely pick the children up to change them. As the date approached for her operation, however, she began to worry not so much about having the implants out as about what to tell the people in her life. Her parents still didn't know she had implants. Neither did her brothers, or most of their closest friends. She told the mothers of the children in her care that she was going to Cleveland for a partial mastecto-my—the same story she told her parents.

Swanson would simply take five days off from work as vacation. But he had to speak to at least one person in the company's benefits department so that his health insurance would pay for the procedure. Initially, the insurance carrier refused to cover the operation, claiming that it was considered cosmetic surgery. Swanson worked closely with Feng to make it clear the operation was hardly cosmetic. Failing to make headway with the company's benefits people, Swanson finally had a no-holds-barred conversation with the insurance carri-er's representative, after which coverage for the explant proce-dure was approved only a week or two before the surgery.

It was a long, agonizing drive—six hours from Midland. After reaching Cleveland, Colleen first went to the Cleveland Clinic for a mammogram, which she then carried with her to Feng's office. On the basis of the examination, Feng recom-mended that she have the implants out immediately. The sur-geon explained the mammogram results which she said, showed that some of Colleen's breast tissue had been destroyed by silicone leaking from her implants. The left breast was much worse than the right, with the breast tissue destroyed down to the rib cage. Indeed, Feng told her, she had just skin over the implant; there was virtually no breast tissue left.

The surgery was set for the next morning. When Colleen Swanson lay on the operating table in Mount Sinai Hospital, Feng had all of three months worth of experience in removing implants. Before the year was out, however, she would perform about 100 of the operations. In 1992, Feng would do as many as 270 explantations and average about 200 more a year thereafter.

When she removes an implant, Feng will typically make a sharp incision under the breast in the area of the original incision. She then uses a knife or scissors to separate the scar tissue around the implant from normal breast tissue, reaching underneath the device to separate it from the muscle. Feng says she usually finds it is easy to separate the scar tissue from the body. It becomes much more difficult when an implant is ruptured and has leaked not only into the muscle but other tissue as well, or when the patient is suffering from severe inflammation. Feng uses ultrasound to help her locate free silicone in the body, though that technique is useful only when silicone has leaked in more than just microscopic amounts. The procedure can take anywhere from one hour for both breasts without reconstruction to as much as four hours when reconstruction from the patient's own body tissue is required or when complications occur.

It would take nearly three hours to undo the operation that Dr. Baker had performed in less than an hour 17 years earlier. Removing breast implants is a far more difficult and invasive operation than putting them in. When a plastic surgeon installs breast implants, they can be folded so that they fit into a small opening, sometimes less than two inches in length. Explantation, however, requires a far larger incision, of up to six inches since the calcified capsule can be extremely hard and inflexible. Patients typically bleed far more during the operation because the surgeon needs to cut deeper to remove the scar tissue.

When Feng cut into Colleen's chest, she found that the implants were oozing silicone gel. The left implant was ruptured and had been for some time. Calcified capsules had formed around the implants to such an extent that the capsules had adhered to the breast tissue itself. The implants had become extremely hard, as firm as softballs. Feng did everything she could to retrieve all of the floating sili-cone inside Colleen, even going deep into the rib cage to scrape it out.

In many cases, the breasts of women who have been explanted return to something close to their preimplanted form in time. Typically, this happens to women who have their implants removed before heavily calcified capsules had formed, which allows them to retain much of their breast tissue. Because Colleen's implants had been in for 17 years and the encapsulation was extreme, Feng had to remove nearly all of her remaining breast tissue.

As Colleen was coming out of the anesthesia in the recovery room, Feng assured her the surgery had gone well. "The first thing I want you to know is that none of this was in your mind," Feng told her. "The implants were leaking and the capsules were very hard."

Colleen left the hospital after a one-day stay, wrapped in bandages from her waist to her collarbone. Two drains were connected to the inside of her chest cavity to collect blood and fluid that flowed from her body to lessen the chance of infection after surgery. The drains hung down to her hips, ending in small, clear plastic bags. John Swanson would empty them every two or three hours, pouring the reddish brown contents into measuring cups to track the amount of fluids leaving Colleen's body. She stayed at the Cleveland Clinic Inn for four days in order to gain enough strength for the return trip to Midland and until Feng could remove the drains.

Despite the nightmare, Colleen felt a sense of revival. "Mentally, I felt like a weight had been lifted off my shoulders," recalls Colleen. "I was relieved, and for the first time the joint pain in my fingers left, within 24 hours of having the implants out. I was happy I had it over with, but I was frightened about how I would look. I began thinking, 'What am I going to look like? What are people going to say? How am I going to handle it?' I felt a lot of anger not just for myself but for all the women who were in the same position as I was."

The return trip was an ordeal—a nearly seven-hour journey under severe physical and emotional duress. She sat in the front seat, which was locked back in a reclining position, a blanket covering her body. Even though she was heavily medicated, pain tore through her chest every time the car hit a bump or made a sharp turn. There was virtually no conversation during the trip. Colleen was mostly crying as Swanson drove home.

Back in Midland, she spent a painful period attempting to recuperate from the surgery. Indeed, just a couple of weeks later, she attended the wedding of her son, Kelly. She shuffled through the ceremony in a haze, her mind clouded by a heavy dose of pain relievers. All through the event, she feared that even the slightest bump would send a new spasm of pain through her chest. She wore a silver-gray dress, one that she had selected several months before the wedding, and one that had required extensive alternation by the time she wore it. She and her daughter, Kathy, stitched protheses into the dress to make it appear that Colleen still had her breasts. Somehow, she survived the trials of an event that should have been one of life's most joyful occasions.

Shortly after the wedding, a Midland couple, not involved with either Dow Chemical or Dow Corning, flew her back to Cleveland in their private plane to have her stitches removed, thinking that she had undergone a partial mastectomy. "They assumed I had cancer and didn't talk about it much," she says. "I told everyone I didn't want to talk about it and they respected that."

But the lie could not hide the anguish the Swansons felt. Colleen would not get a glimpse of what she looked like until she unwrapped the bandages on her body a full month after the surgery in late July 1991. She chose to go through this tribulation alone, in the privacy of their master bedroom, when her husband was at work. Swanson would not even know his wife had removed her bandages until he returned home that evening. And she wouldn't show him the result of the surgery until just before they went to bed.

For weeks, he had braced himself for the worst. "I knew she was going to look bad," says Swanson. "Dr. Feng had told me pretty much what to expect, and she might have been a little more candid or blunt with me than with Colleen. She said she had to take everything out."

So when Colleen took off her blouse and showed him her

chest, he was not shocked or surprised by what he saw. Indeed, his first remark was an unusual one, something to break the tension of the moment, something to draw a smile from his wife and assure her that it made little difference to him. There hadn't been much humor in their lives for a long time. Swanson wanted to somehow change that, even at this awkward and painful time.

"Va-va voom," he joked, at his very first glimpse of her body. "Dr. Feng did a marvelous job, Colleen. The incision is healing up well."

Then, he took his wife in his arms and kissed her as she cried and cried.

Swanson had steeled himself for this moment. He had convinced himself that at this point Colleen's physical appearance was almost trivial. He had told himself that it really didn't matter that his wife would be without breasts for the rest of her life. What mattered was that they would have another chance at living a good life together. "Whatever I had felt in the past about the importance of the female breast was by that time a memory," he recalls. "Her breasts were not cosmetically or sexually important to either one of us. The removal of her breasts was what we believed to be a life-prolonging necessity. This was going to give her a chance at hopefully regaining a more healthy life, and this was going to give us a chance to regain the quality of life we had lost over the past six or seven years."

Though she would often cry—even years later—when she looked at herself in the mirror, Colleen could at least feel great relief at her husband's acceptance of her appearance. "I would have been very happy if I could have gone the rest of my life without John seeing it," says Colleen. "But he was so good about it. He never made me feel ashamed. He knew I was devastated by it, but he never made me feel ashamed or uncomfortable. He showed me that a woman can live and enjoy life without breasts. Women do not need breasts to be complete and whole."

There were practical problems, of course, such as finding clothes to wear. But eventually, once the wounds on her chest had healed, she would wear prostheses or a fully padded bra held to the chest with metal stays. In spite of her ravaged chest, Colleen never once wavered in her belief that she had made the right decision to have the implants out. She was glad they were gone. She believed the operation may well have saved her life. It had certainly, in her mind, prolonged it.

*   *   *

Less than two weeks after Colleen's surgery in Cleveland, Dow Corning shipped several cardboard boxes stuffed with tens of thousands of documents to the FDA offices in Washington in hopes of proving that its implants were safe. The company waited until the day before the last filing deadline on July 8 to ship the randomly organized information to the agency in support of its "premarket approval application" (PMAA) to keep the devices on the market. Dow Corning was one of four implant makers to seek FDA approval. Surgitek, now a subsidiary of Bristol-Myers Squibb, decided to withdraw from the business altogether, saying it was unable to meet a 90-day deadline for the information set by the government.

Together, the four companies remaining in the silicone breast implant business—Bioplasty Incorporated, Dow Corning, McGhan Medical, and Mentor Corporation—filed so much documentation that it filled 15 large file boxes. Dow Corning's submission was, by far, the biggest—in part because all the other companies used Dow Corning silicone in their implants. So virtually all the safety data on silicone had to come from Dow Corning, which submitted over 30 years of test results to the FDA.

Little more than a month later, on August 12, the head of the FDA's Breast Prosthesis task force issued a scathing review of Dow Corning's clinical studies, stating that they were "so weak that they cannot provide a reasonable assurance of the safety and effectiveness of these devices." He noted that the studies "provide no assurance that the full range of complications are included, no dependable measure of the incidence of complications, no reliable measure of the revision rate, and no quantitative measure of patient benefit.... [Surgeons surveyed were instructed] to report only complications associated with the implant. As a result, the only complications reported are those at the implant site. This prevents these investigations from detecting systemic adverse effects.... [This] causes an underestimate of both the types and incidence of complications."

Still, the company had sent its boxes of documents to Washington regulators with much confidence and fanfare, even issuing a press release on the filing. Burson Marstellar, the pricey doyen of the public relations world, prepared a long memo for Dow Corning executives to help them answer expected questions from reporters. The public relations experts, who would at one point reportedly bill the company nearly $1 million a month for their services, drafted 71 potential questions and carefully worded answers for executives.

Some of the proposed replies were nearly silly. One example:

QUESTION: "Isn't this just a public relations ploy?"

ANSWER: "It's nothing of the kind. This is a significant step."

Other questions focused on the history of litigation surrounding implants. At least one left even Burson Marstellar's pros at a loss for an answer.

QUESTION: "If implants are safe, why are you settling lawsuits lodged against you rather than fighting them in court?"

ANSWER: "We sometimes settle lawsuits because it makes good economic sense to do so. That has nothing to do with implant safety."

QUESTION: "But in the 1984 Stern case, the judge found that the evidence showed your implant was inherently defective, and the court awarded the plaintiff $1.5 million in punitive damages. You were found guilty of fraud, and the judge concluded your actions were 'highly reprehensible.' Is this a company people can trust?"

"(Need response)."

THE LITTLE CANDY STORE ACROSS THE STREET GETS A NEW BOSS

The pains started in her feet. A piercing, inexplicable pain attacked the joints of Mariann Hopkins's feet, forcing her to give up her daily three-mile run. Then, the hurt traveled to her hands, turning her fingers purple. Finally, it racked many of the joints in her 5-foot-3-inch body.

For Hopkins, an administrative assistant at California's Sonoma State University, the ordeal began in 1973, when, at the age of 27, she discovered a lump in her breast. She had been married nearly 10 years to Richard, a San Francisco fireman, and already had two sons—Mark, 9, and Tim, 7. Within three years, Hopkins had lost both her breasts because of precancerous tissue.

Silicone breast implants, her doctor assured her, were a safe and viable alternative to a flat chest. "The doctor did tell me there was a rare possibility I could get an infection or my blood might not circulate properly," she recalls. Yet six weeks after her Dow Corning implants were put into place, she developed severe complications. The left implant began to push its way out of her body, causing her left breast to turn black until the skin died. The surgeon grafted skin from her stomach onto the opening in her chest and six months later installed a new set of implants.

Within a year, however, her feet began to ache. "I was having difficulty completing my three-mile run," Hopkins says. "At first, it felt as if my shoes were too tight and my feet would just hurt. I bought new running shoes, but it didn't solve the problem. Then, my knees would hurt and I found myself out of breath. I just couldn't complete three miles anymore, and it wasn't because I was out of shape. I had been running for a couple of years." She began to feel more joint pain, then fatigue and muscle spasms. After her fingers turned purple in late 1977, she was diagnosed with mixed-connective-tissue disease. The diagnosis meant that she suffered from a combination of auto-immune diseases. In her case, it was lupus, scleroderma, and polymyositis (inflammation of the muscles). One doctor prescribed steroids and anti-inflammatory drugs, then muscle relaxants and antidepressants. No one, however, linked her health problems to the implants in her chest. "I saw my plastic surgeon regularly," she says. "My breasts never got hard and they never hurt. The doctors said a woman shouldn't worry if she's not having any problems. I believed that to be true."

It wasn't until 1986—a full decade after she got implants—that her plastic surgeon discovered her first rupture. It took surgeons five hours to remove the silicone that had leaked out of the implant from her body—and even then they couldn't recapture all of the chemical. And then her doctor replaced the implants with another set of Dow Corning models. Still more complications caused a third and fourth set of implants to be installed in 1986.

Two years later, when the FDA held hearings on implants in November 1988, she saw Dan Bolton, the attorney who had helped win the $1.7 million judgment for Maria Stern in 1984, on TV commenting on the potential health hazards of silicone. "Before then, I really didn't think that anyone ever had a problem with implants," she says. "My plastic surgeon told me he only had seen one other patient with problems and she had been accidentally hit in the chest. Finally, I learned I wasn't the only one out there, and I learned that Dow Corning had been sued before because of their implants."

Hopkins filed her lawsuit against the company on

December 1, 1988. Just before the trial was set to begin in June 1991, her physician discovered that silicone had leaked into her breast cavity, her right shoulder, and her right arm. He recommended that her implants be removed for good. They were flat. It took UCLA surgeon William Shaw, Lu-Jean Feng's old mentor, 11 hours to carve them out of her body, collect still more leaking silicone, and reconstruct her breasts with skin grafts from thigh tissue. Three days later, Hopkins developed a blood clot under her right arm and found herself undergoing yet another terrifying trauma: Doctors laid five leeches on the site of her blood clot to suck her blood for one and one-half hours. "I know they lanced me," she said. "I didn't know they had the leeches on until I saw one in my doctor's hand and almost passed out." Hopkins was then given a shot of morphine to calm her before she went into surgery again.

When the trial finally began in October, the jury hearing her lawsuit—which alleged that Dow Corning sold a defective product and withheld important safety information from patients—saw an emaciated woman in the courtroom. Once an avid runner who liked to paint and nurture orchids, Hopkins claimed that health problems resulting from her implants had caused her weight to drop to just 98 pounds from 120. When she wasn't holding onto her husband for support, she walked slowly with a cane. "You weren't going to find a more compelling plaintiff than Hopkins," says Dan Bolton, who represented her. "She was married. She had a family. She had no pre-existing psychological problems. She also had implants for reconstruction, not for cosmetic reasons. Some jurors will look at a plaintiff who had cosmetic surgery and think that she really didn't need the operation so now she has to suffer the consequences. That was not true in the Hopkins case."

This time, however, Dow Corning's defense was far more organized than it had been in the Stern case. Frank Woodside III, a lawyer-physician based in Cincinnati, led Dow Corning's defense team. He had spent the past dozen years defending Bendectin, the morning-sickness pill that Merrill-Dow had taken off the market because it allegedly caused birth defects in the children of women who took it. Woodside tried to keep many of the most damaging documents from Dow Corning's files from surfacing, on the basis that they were either not relevant to the case or not authentic. He called to the stand experts on behalf of the company who were far less hostile and combative than those in the Stern case.

Ultimately, however, Woodside failed to prevent the jury from seeing the Dow Corning internal memos that raised significant questions about the product's safety. And although the company's expert testimony was far more competent than it had been in the Stern trial, it still was not convincing enough for the jury. "Dow's experts were a little more uptight, not as casual and not as conversant with the jury," believes Bolton. "They were a little too academic and didactic."

For a weary Hopkins, sitting in the courtroom absorbing all the testimony, it was a devastating experience. "Even though Dan told me about the memos and the company's own research that showed that silicone could be reactive, it was hard to sit there and watch it all unfold before me," she remembers. "At the time, I would have preferred that it not be true because it was so difficult to think that a company could place so little value on a person's life. It was shocking to sit there and hear Dow Corning's own memos and own research convict them. It wasn't what the attorneys alleged or what I said. They convicted themselves."

Just before the jury convened, Dow Corning offered Hopkins $200,000 to settle out of court, according to Bolton. She refused. On December 13, 1991, the jury awarded Hopkins $7.3 million—at the time the largest victory ever for a plaintiff in a breast implant suit. The jury not only found the company's breast implants defective, it also found Dow Corning guilty of fraud. Hopkins's attorneys argued that the internal company documents suggested that Dow Corning had covered up evidence of possible dangers and discouraged its scientists from researching them.

The decision had the force of a detonating bomb on Dow Corning. The company's executives could not understand how the jury could award $7.3 million to Hopkins when two of her doctors—called by Dow Corning as witnesses—testified that some symptoms of her connective-tissue disease preceded her breast implant surgery. Some of the company's executives arrogantly believed they lost the case not because of the merits of Hopkins's allegations but because she was a highly sympathetic plaintiff. "The jury felt sorry for her," says one key Dow Corning executive. "The judge limited the number of experts to one or two on each side or issue. The jury had a hard time figuring out which expert to believe and didn't have the scientific background to evaluate the testimony. So the jury felt sorry for Hopkins and ruled in her favor."

So incredulous and shell-shocked was the company's management at the Hopkins loss that it approved a communications department press release headed "Dow Corning and its employees call San Francisco jury award regarding breast implants outrageous; Characterize breast implant debate as sensationalistic and politicized." The document is notable for its strident denunciation of both the verdict and the increasingly negative media coverage of the implant issue. Rylee, whose off-handed remarks had publicly embarrassed the company in the *Business Week* story six months earlier, was not quoted in the release.

Instead, the company produced Swanson's friend, Dan Hayes, the chief executive and president of Dow Corning Wright. Prompted by the company's PR consultants, Hayes's comments sounded more like a tirade than the cautious remarks typical of most corporate executives and Hayes in particular. At no time did he express any concern for Hopkins or any other women who believed their health problems were caused by breast implants. He declared:

> This jury verdict symbolizes the politicization of the entire breast implant issue. Thirty years of scientific data is being ignored because of the sensational media environment that has been established by plaintiff's attorneys who stand to make a lot of money from these awards. It's no wonder a jury can ignore the science when some media serve up sensational tabloid journalism like the Connie Chung show, and

rehash the same one-sided, inflammatory claims about breast implants made by Phil Donahue—while the FDA is making a final determination concerning the future availability of this important product....

Not only is it difficult for a jury to make a decision but it is virtually impossible for women to make an informed choice about breast implants, when the inaccurate and sensational side of this story so dominates the media. It is clear that the deck is stacked against women across this country who value and want access to this product. The process for determining the safety and the public health need of breast implants has been destroyed, and as a science based company, we must register our total disgust with this entire process.

Dow Corning then called the verdict "an affront" to its more than 8000 employees. But there was at least one employee at headquarters who thought it was an affront for the company to say that he was outraged by the jury's verdict. If anything, John Swanson was outraged that the company would presume to speak for him. "I thought the verdict was legitimate," he recalls, "and ultimately, all of the company's appeals including the final one to the United States Supreme Court would uphold its legitimacy. The company's reaction was the epitome of stridency, arrogance, and outrageousness. It was an example of crisis management at its worst."

He believed the news release was also further proof that the company had no coherent public relations strategy other than its willingness to react defensively and arrogantly to each new allegation. Nearly every day, the company would issue—either through a company spokesperson, a Reed Committee member, or a news release—yet another belligerent remark or comment that never expressed any concern for women with silicone implants. Robert Grupp, the manager of external communications, who was now fielding phone calls from all over the country, told one journalist the company would not discuss its safety studies with reporters who had "no scientific credentials."

Whether it was a newly filed lawsuit, another demand from the FDA for more information, or new charges in newspaper reports based on "leaked" documents from the Hopkins case, the company seemed prepared simply to crank out a press release to refute it.

By late 1991, with events obviously spinning out of control, a small cadre of public relations operatives from the Chicago office of Burson Marstellar had taken up residence in Dow Corning's communications department to work more closely with Barbara S. Carmichael, United States area vice-president of communications, and Grupp.

The almost daily dose of negative news virtually paralyzed the senior executive team. The headlines in newspapers around the world provided ample evidence of the building pressure: "Breast Implant Maker Accused on Data." "Memos: Employees Sought Inquiry into Implant Safety." "United States Authorities May Order Halt to $400 Million Breast Implant Industry." "As Silicone Issue Grows Women Take Agony and Anger to Court." "Liability Problems Seen for Corning, Dow Chemical in Implant Controversy."

Chairman Jack Ludington, who had spent years building Dow Corning's reputation as a worldly and highly ethical corporation, now watched his work come apart. Dow Corning was so pivotal to his life that Ludington's idea of a good weekend was showing up for work on Saturday morning at 10. His wife had created a small social life for him in Midland, but he had few, if any, hobbies or outside interests. The one-time missionary for the corporation's code of ethics and high-minded values found himself powerless to reverse the disastrous slide in Dow Corning's reputation.

Yet both he and Chief Executive Larry Reed still refused to publicly comment or become involved in any visible way with the controversy. "Reed was kind of lost," recalls Gordon C. Britton, then editor of the *Midland Daily News*. "He insulated himself. He was uncomfortable with the press. He was the kind of guy who liked to come in, shake your hand and get out as fast as he could." Even Reed's appearances for lunch in the company cafeteria—once a fairly regular occurence—became less frequent. He would sometimes walk briskly through the cafeteria, his eyes avoiding everyone who saw him, to grab a sandwich and head straight back to his office. Other times, he would schedule noon-time meetings in his office, with lunch sent in. As the company reeled from the incessant barrage of negative publicity, some employees began asking, "Where's Larry?"

Some of the company's media advisors were asking the same question. "When the big flap hit, Reed and the other senior executives around him literally went into the bunker," recalls Arnold Zenker, the consultant who advised Dow Corning executives on media training. "I would go out there with Burson Marstellar and we would sit in one room and they would be hidden in the executive chambers. We never had much contact with them. It was the goddamnest thing I had ever seen. We were with some of the external communications staff like Bob Grupp and messages were nearly conveyed by smoke signal. You'd fly out of there and never see Reed and his senior people. They were shell shocked. How do you compete with women saying they were destroyed by these mean men in Midland, Michigan?"

At one point, Zenker was so frustrated by the experience that he wrote a letter to the company trying to explain that there was no reason to continue to fight the fight. "It made no difference if they were right or wrong," recalls Zenker. "No one was going to pull them out of it. It had developed a force of its own, and no way could they pull out of the slide."

So remote was Reed that he had delegated basic responsibility for managing the controversy to J. Kerm Campbell, who now effectively chaired the Reed Committee. Campbell, in turn, had transferred the job of public spokesperson to Rylee, Hayes, Bob Grupp, and others. Exactly what anyone could say was often controlled by Jenkins, the general counsel, who favored saying as little as possible, a tactic that was eroding the company's reputation in the media.

When a reporter for *The New York Times* wrote an article critical of the company's public relations mistakes in managing the crisis, no one in the communications department wanted to bring the story to Reed's attention. The article, which appeared on January 29, 1992, reported that Dow Corning's mistakes included the lack of public action by Reed, the company's failure to express sympathy and support for women who said they were harmed by implants, and its failure to get the worst news out quickly. "Mr. Reed's actions in particular call to mind the aloofness of Exxon's chief executive, Lawrence Rawl, during the early stages of the *Valdez* spill—a marked contrast to the public leadership demonstrated by Johnson & Johnson's chairman, James Burke, following the discovery of poison-laced Tylenol capsules in 1983," said the *Times*. When Reed finally read the article at his desk, at least one employee overheard him utter the word "aloof?"—apparently incredulous that anyone could think he was detached from the crisis.

The PR advisors also found themselves up against an entrenched legal machine. Ever since the company had lost the Stern case in 1984, Dow Corning seemed to have become nearly paranoid about its legal vulnerability. Decisions related in even the remotest way to the company's breast implant operations were almost always made or approved by the company's legal department. Under General Counsel Jenkins, the legal group had become the company's fastest growing department. In addition to a bulging permanent staff on the second floor of DC-1, Dow Corning had contracted with more than 180 outside attorneys by early 1992 to help in the defense of breast implants.

Clearly, the influence of the legal department was increasing as the implant controversy heated up. Jenkins also was taking a more dominant leadership position on the company's Reed Committee. Kerm Campbell had now been commissioned by Reed as the company's overall implant czar. His overriding challenge was to manage Dow Corning through the crisis. Though not known as a strong-willed or decisive executive, Campbell was highly admired for his people skills. He had the reputation for being the kind of manager who led by consensus, who wasn't always willing to fight for his own position unless there was little chance of losing. "Campbell could have been a diplomat," says one observer who thought highly of the executive. "It was not his personality to get angry, lose his temper, or stand up and pound on a table."

In contrast, Jenkins—who emerged as one of the key hardliners on the breast implant issue—had a far more dominant personality. He was an imposingly tall, intelligent man who did not hesitate to take a strong stand and fight for it—even if it meant intimidating some of his Dow Corning colleagues. Always well-dressed and highly articulate, he inspired confidence. "Jim was the kind of guy who was always telling people 'There's no problem. Don't worry about it. It's just not an issue,'" recalls an adviser to the company. "Unfortunately, too many lawyers were making too many decisions. Had Campbell played a more active role, I think things would have been different."

Jenkins convinced Chairman Ludington and others not to disclose many of the documents that surfaced in the Stern and Hopkins cases when Campbell and some other Reed Committee members believed it was no longer viable to maintain the company's stonewalling tactics. "Jim is the one who pushed Jack into the hardball position," concedes one insider. "Jim was wrong about that. He created a lot of the problems."

Jenkins also kept many of the most damaging memos and documents from the senior team managing the crisis—ostensibly to protect the company from having its key executives dragged into litigation. If they hadn't seen or weren't aware of the memos, they couldn't possibly be expected to answer questions about them from plaintiff's attorneys. Thus, they were unaware of marketing manager Chuck Leach's "crossed-fingers" memo and of the so-called "Pinto" memo from the sales rep who warned he was losing customers because they were disenchanted with the quality of Dow Corning implants. As a consequence, many of the people trying to manage the company through the controversy had little idea of how those documents cast Dow Corning in such a negative light. Indeed, several top executives saw and read some of the documents for the first time in newspapers. "Some of us had no idea that a lot of that crap was in the files," says an insider.

Thanks largely to the company's aggressively combative strategy, Dow Corning was acquiring the image of a careless and heartless corporation.

*   *   *

From the day of the Hopkins verdict, the company found itself under continuous assault—from contingency-fee lawyers, consumer advocates, federal regulators, reporters, and angry women who blamed any number of illnesses on their breast implants. When the Hopkins decision came in, some 137 suits were pending against the company for health-care claims. That number would grow to 3558 by the end of 1992 and to more than 12,000 by the end of 1993. Sidney Wolfe's Public Citizen Health Research Group had begun selling a "how-to-sue-a-manufacturer kit" to lawyers for $750 each. Trial lawyers began advertising in newspapers, seeking implanted women eager to file lawsuits against Dow Corning or other implant makers. One Texas law firm lured potential clients with the advertising line, "Are 'dream breasts' to die for?" Attorney Dan Bolton alone received close to 1000 phone calls from women with implants within six months of the Hopkins decision. About 100 of them resulted in lawsuits.

Even worse for Dow Corning, the loss in the Hopkins case led to a flurry of highly critical stories in the media. "It was sound-bite hell," says Barbara Carmichael who handled many of the calls at Dow Corning. Some of the most damaging reporting came from an enterprising reporter who had covered the Hopkins trial for *The San Francisco Examiner*. Seth Rosenfeld sat in the courtroom nearly every day of the trial, taking copious notes on the testimony and the documents entered into evidence. Bolton leaked some of the memos to Rosenfeld, who sent them to Dr. Norman D. Anderson, then a member of the FDA's advisory panel and a high-profile critic of breast implants. Anderson personally delivered the documents to FDA Commissioner David Kessler's home on January 3, 1992.

The documents raised significant doubts about the safety of Dow Corning's silicone breast implants. Many of them—dubbed "screamer memos" by Carmichael because of the attention they received—had been seen by attorney Bolton nine years earlier, when he had sat for a week in a large, cold

room at the company's headquarters surrounded by 200 unla-
beled boxes of data. Since then, some three-quarters of a million women had received silicone breast implants without having access to much of the information Bolton had unearthed.
Some of the documents that reported the results of internal
studies suggested that over the past 25 years Dow Corning
had reason to believe at the very least that immune systems
could be affected by silicone. A 1974 study—which had surfaced in the Hopkins trial—had been performed by Dow
Corning to determine whether different silicone compounds
had commercial potential as an "adjuvant," a substance that
could heighten or prolong immune response to other materials. The 10-month study on guinea pigs found that one version of silicone fluid used in breast implants increased
immune response tenfold when compared to implants filled
with saline solution. Robert LeVier, a coauthor of the 1974
study and still a key player in the implant debate, then wrote:
"We have data showing that organosilicon compounds (silicone) can stimulate the immune response."

LeVier would dismiss the restricted study on January 17,
1992, calling it "uninteresting" because, he claimed, more
recent, state-of-the-art studies showed silicone had no
immune effects. He told one reporter it was "ridiculous" to
suggest that the study proved that silicone might affect
women's immune systems. In fact, he argued, it was merely a
"screen," not a definitive study. But a 1985 memo by LeVier's
coauthor, William F. Boley, seemed to suggest otherwise. "I
think we probably should start at least acknowledging the
potential for sensitization," he wrote. Boley called for further
testing after warning that a particular formulation of the gel
could cause cancer. Without additional studies, he argued, "I
think we have excessive personal and corporate liability exposure." It would be several more years, however, before Boley's
warnings would be acted upon by the company.

The package of documents Kessler reviewed also contained
a 1967 study in which liquid silicone was injected into 11
dogs. Three of the injected animals developed inflammation of
the thyroid. A year later, another Dow Corning study in which

various silicone materials were implanted in 35 beagles showed that four of them developed the same problem. None of the control dogs, which did not receive silicone, suffered the condition. Other studies—performed outside and received by Dow Corning in 1970 and 1972—showed that liquid silicone, when injected into laboratory rats and mice, could move into their immune systems.

Nonetheless, LeVier was correct in saying that later studies conducted by Dow Corning concluded that silicone did not activate the immune system. But those results were deemed virtually meaningless by UCLA scientist Nir Kossovsky, who had testified in the Hopkins trial and who also was a consultant to the FDA advisory panel. Kossovsky believed that Dow Corning failed to follow the routine scientific procedure of having a control group with which to compare results.

Other leaked documents were nonscientific memos from Dow Corning salesmen and plastic surgeons who had significant complaints about the company's products. Among them were the letters of Dr. Charles Vinnik, a prominent plastic surgeon in Las Vegas, who had complained frequently about the company's breast implants. In one letter, Vinnik claimed he felt "like a broken record" but that the company had done little to follow up on his complaints. He told of an incident in which a Dow Corning implant had ruptured and spilled its contents—which he described as having the "consistency of 50 weight motor oil"—onto his operating room floor.

Three days after receiving the documents, on January 6, 1992, Kessler called for a 45-day moratorium on all sales of silicone gel breast implants pending further study of their safety. Alarmed by the contents of the memos, he also recalled the FDA advisory panel to consider new evidence. Dr. Norman Cole, president of the American Society of Plastic and Reconstructive Surgeons, called Kessler's action "unconscionable—an outrage." Cole believed the moratorium "created hysteria, anxiety and panic" among women with implants and demanded that Kessler change the members of the FDA's advisory panel because, Cole claimed, they were unqualified to judge the safety of the implants. "Patients and physicians alike deserve to have such an important ruling made on the basis of a thorough, expert, scientific evaluation," charged Cole. "Such an analysis cannot be provided by a panel whose voting members include only one epidemiologist and no rheumatologists."

Cole later arranged to call Kessler's boss, Health and Human Services Secretary Louis Sullivan, on at least two occasions to urge him to intervene and replace the FDA advisory board members with a new panel of more highly credentialed scientists. He sent letters to 50,000 surgeons asking them to "write, call or fax" Sullivan and demand that he remove Kessler from the process. Cole included Sullivan's address, his phone number, and his office fax number. Many surgeons responded with letters that urged Sullivan to fire Kessler from his job.

Dow Corning quickly supported Cole's demands with yet another press release loaded with highly combative language. "We recognize that our detractors, including special interest groups and their friends in the plaintiff's bar, are opposed to real experts getting involved in this debate," charged Hayes, who continued to believe that Kessler's decision was politically motivated. "After all, they cannot win when true science is the basis for the discussion."

To some degree, of course, Hayes was right. The issue was becoming increasingly politicized—but not only because of consumer advocates and contingency-fee attorneys. It also was becoming a political issue because of the plastic surgeons and corporate lobbyists who were applying formidable pressure to keep implants on the market and to attack those who threatened the viability of what had become a $300 million business for plastic surgeons in the United States.

Indeed, when the FDA advisory panel met in October 1991, the plastic surgeons paid to fly nearly 400 women to Washington to visit senators and representatives to talk up the benefits of implants in helping to restore their self-esteem. The surgeons, their nurses, and satisfied patients also flooded Congress and the FDA with more than 20,000 letters urging that implants be left on the market.

Among other things, they charged that several of the members of the FDA advisory panel had obvious conflicts of interest. Marc A. Lappe, the University of Illinois professor whose devastating testimony in both the Stern and Hopkins cases had severely harmed Dow Corning, was an FDA panelist. Yet, he was receiving between $75,000 and $150,000 annually as an expert witness for plaintiffs in breast implant cases. Another panelist, psychologist Rita Freedman, had written that breast implants perpetuate what she called "the myth of Barbie Doll's body."

Under severe pressure, Kessler agreed to name two rheumatologists as consultants to the FDA advisory panel to help it more effectively evaluate the claims that silicone could cause auto-immune diseases. He also took away the voting rights of one board member, Norman Anderson, who had brought the Hopkins documents to his attention, on the grounds that he had prejudged the case by publicly denouncing implants.

Kessler, who had become commissioner of the FDA just a few months earlier, was subjected to continual personal and professional pressure. At one point, his wife, Paulette, was called at home by a lobbying consultant for the plastic surgeons. The consultant, Nancy Taylor, asked Kessler's wife if she had silicone breast implants and whether her husband was cracking down on them because she experienced problems with the implants. Taylor contended that she was only trying to help a reporter confirm or dismiss the rumor. Mrs. Kessler emphatically denied she had implants, but a few weeks later, Commissioner Kessler received a telephone call from another reporter. This time, the journalist asked if Paulette Kessler had ruptured one of her silicone implants in a skiing accident in Colorado. The reporter claimed he was checking a story given to him by a plastic surgeon. Kessler kept the story from surfacing by explaining that his wife did not ski.

The incidents showed just how vicious the lobbying campaign to keep implants on the market had become. Cole would later deny that the American Society of Plastic and Reconstructive Surgeons orchestrated the rumor campaign to build a case that Kessler had a personal bias on the issue. But Cole acknowledged to one reporter that he had heard of at least one plastic surgeon who actually checked his patient records on a woman named Kessler, thinking she might be the commissioner's wife. Cole's group also hired two of Commissioner Kessler's closest friends—an attorney with whom Kessler had worked when he was an aide to Senator Orrin Hatch in the early 1980s and a former FDA official with whom he had co-authored medical articles—to help lobby on behalf of the plastic surgeons. It also hired several other high-powered Washington lobbyists with connections to Sullivan, Kessler's boss, and others in the Bush administration.

*   *   *

After Kessler's January 6, 1992, moratorium, Dow Corning's board of directors began to focus on successors to both Dow Corning Chairman Ludington and Chief Executive Reed. Neither executive seemed either willing or capable of leading the company through the breast implant controversy, and there were few signs that the worst was yet over. The company had already shut down its implant production lines in Hemlock, Michigan, and, Arlington, Tennessee, after the FDA moratorium. It had announced on January 14 that it was taking a $25 million pretax charge to earnings for costs due to the controversy. Before the end of January, Dow Corning also had hired former United States Attorney General Griffin B. Bell's Atlanta-based law firm, King and Spalding, to conduct an independent investigation of the company's behavior in making, selling, and testing breast implants. Bell had developed a reputation for objectively investigating corporate crises. His firm, for example, had investigated E. F. Hutton's check-kiting scam as well as Exxon Corporation's highly publicized *Valdez* oil spill off the coast of Alaska.

The most qualified person to take charge was Keith R. McKennon, an affable executive vice-president of Dow Corning's parent, Dow Chemical. As a Dow Corning director, he was well aware of the mounting problems the company was facing. He knew the company's senior management team, and he had been privy to many of the key decisions leading up to the crisis. Even more important, McKennon was a master image maker. Over the years, he had shown enough public relations acumen to earn the nickname of "the fireman" for his ability to extinguish huge blazes of negative publicity.

In the mid-1970s, he had entered the public affairs arena for Dow, whose public reputation had been badly tarnished by the Agent Orange and dioxin controversies. McKennon had also been involved in handling the controversy over Bendectin, the morning sickness pill made by Merrill-Dow that allegedly resulted in birth defects.

On the advice of his father, an Oregon farmer, McKennon had joined Dow Chemical in 1955, after earning a degree in agricultural chemistry from Oregon State University. His father had heard about the joint venture between Dow and Corning that was already producing silicones, and he thought the product had great promise. "In a way, I got to Dow because it had just formed Dow Corning," McKennon says. He landed a job in Dow's research and development department and became a business manager in 1968. But he made an unusual detour into the public affairs function in the mid-1970s that helped propel him to still higher levels of responsibility within the company.

McKennon fostered productive relationships with legislators, the media, and the public, winning immediate credibility with his no-nonsense comments and his easy accessibility. At first blush, McKennon is one of those rare executives who seems to almost relish a good challenge. During interviews, he nearly invites probing questions with the words "Fire away." His informal style is disarming.

The first Dow Corning director to approach McKennon about the possibility of a move was Van Campbell, the chief financial officer of Corning. The company was reeling from both the Hopkins verdict and the FDA moratorium. Campbell told McKennon that his background and experience made him an ideal candidate to take over the top job at Dow Corning.

Campbell said it would please him and other board members if McKennon would consider making the change.

McKennon, who was then 57 years old and had suffered from a form of cancer, non-Hodgkin's lymphoma, was looking forward to retiring to his home on the Oregon coast where, as he has put it, he can hear the bark of the seals and the crashing of the waves on the beach. McKennon didn't decline the job outright, but he made it clear that his first choice was "to retire with dignity from the Dow Chemical Company and go live the rest of my life." Soon, however, McKennon was receiving overtures from other directors, including Enrique Falla, the chief financial officer of Dow Chemical, as well as the chairmen and chief executives of Dow and Corning.

At the very least, McKennon felt he needed to have the title of chief executive officer to effectively deal with the crisis. McKennon already knew all the senior executives at Dow Corning, because he had been one of the 15 directors on its board since December 1987. He also had met Dan Hayes when McKennon's son dated Hayes's daughter in the 1970s.

McKennon would later say he accepted the challenge out of loyalty to Dow Chemical. "I did it because a company I owe everything to asked me to," he said. "You kind of get attached after 37 years." McKennon said he would move if given the same base salary he had at Dow and if the retirement benefits he had accrued at Dow not be penalized by the transfer. The company ensured that McKennon's retirement benefits from Dow Chemical began as soon as he switched jobs. He also asked to bring with him Dr. Ralph Cook, a Dow Chemical official who had worked with him on the Agent Orange crisis, and arranged a $100,000 bonus to entice Cook to Dow Corning as head of epidemiology to oversee any and all new research on silicones.

Once the details of his compensation package and retirement benefits were nailed down, McKennon retired from Dow Chemical on February 7 with the understanding that he would become chief executive of Dow Corning if approved by the board. Three days later, Dow Corning's board of directors met via a telephone conference call to make it official. McKennon then moved from his office at 2030 Dow Center in Midland to Dow Corning's corporate center five miles away.

Shortly before the announcement on February 10, Reed was summoned to Dow Chemical's private hangar at the Tri-Cities Airport by Jamie Houghton and Frank Popoff, chief executive officers of Corning Incorporated and Dow Chemical, respectively. Neither Houghton nor Popoff thought Reed had managed the crisis effectively. Later, with reporters from chemical trade magazines in the room, Popoff would issue an extraordinary public rebuke. Reed, he said, "was not emotionally equipped to handle the controversy. When the safety of implants became an issue, the company should have been in the first phase of damage control rather than the first phase of denial."

But first, in a conference room at the Dow hangar, the two parent company CEOs told Reed he was being stripped of the chief executive title he had held since 1988. Ludington would retire as chairman, but be given the honorary title of chairman emeritus to take some of the sting out of the ouster. McKennon would then assume the chairman and chief executive titles, while Reed would remain as president—the job he had held since 1984—and gain the title of chief operating officer. He would report directly to McKennon. The management shakeup—although long overdue—surprised most of the executives at Dow Corning.

Meanwhile, after a long, torturous internal debate, three of the key members of the Reed Committee had just decided to disclose publicly the safety tests on silicone and other documents the company had long fought to protect. "Some people inside the corporation thought we shouldn't do it," recalls Rylee. "We shouldn't let anyone force us into releasing the data. Instead, we should continue to take a hard line. But we were getting killed in the media. People were accusing us of being secretive. "

On January 20, the FDA had asked Dow Corning to make public many key documents on implants so that women and their doctors could evaluate the evidence for themselves. Two days later, the company had released a group of scientific studies. Now, it was about to disclose several hundred additional pages of internal documents, the size of two fat phonebooks. By this time even Jenkins had to agree with Campbell and Rylee that it was necessary to get the information.

The next morning, on February 10, Rylee announced the document disclosure on national television in an interview with Harry Smith of the CBS *This Morning* show from a Memphis studio. Then he boarded a chartered Lear jet to fly him to Washington, D.C., where he was scheduled to do a noon press conference with reporters at the Washington Press Club.

As Rylee was en route to Washington, he received a telephone call from Ludington, who was apparently unaware of the impending management changes. The Dow Corning chairman had heard of the decision to release the information and was angry about it. He insisted that Rylee refuse to disclose the documents.

"Jack," Rylee said, "I already said on national television I would do it."

"Well, tell them you've changed your mind," insisted Ludington.

"I can't do that. I'm either going to release all of this at the press club or I am going to have to resign from the company because my credibility is at stake."

Reluctantly, Ludington agreed that the company now had no choice. The company could not withstand the abrupt resignation of Rylee—especially if it ever became known why he was quitting. So Rylee appeared before a crowded room of reporters at the Washington Press Club and made it official: Dow Corning would finally release the results of confidential biosafety documents that had never before been made public.

Rylee was planning to return to Memphis after the press conference, but he received an urgent phone call at the Willard Hotel where he was staying. He was instructed to fly immediately to Midland and go straight to Dow Chemical headquarters to meet with McKennon.

"What's the deal?" he asked.

"Just do it," Rylee was told. "All of this will become clear when you do."

When he arrived at the corporate hangar in Midland, a car was waiting to drive him to Dow Chemical's "pink palace." As soon as Rylee walked into McKennon's office, he heard the executive say, "I'm your new boss."

"SELL THE SUCKER"

John Swanson knew it would not be easy, but he also knew he could wait no longer. They had been good friends, close friends for nearly two decades. Yet Dan Hayes, the chief executive of the Dow Corning subsidiary that made and sold breast implants, still didn't know about Colleen's travails or his friend's decision to recuse himself from the issue. Hayes, however, was coming to visit Swanson in Midland in early February 1992, and Swanson finally decided to tell his friend everything.

For years, he and Dan Hayes had been golfing buddies in the annual three-day invitational tournament at the Midland Country Club in August. Indeed, only six months earlier, the pair had finished in second place in the 1991 contest when Swanson, in natty blue knickers and a white Kangol cap, sunk a 34-foot putt on the 18th hole of the final round. Hayes and his wife, who lived in Memphis, would almost always stay with the Swansons in their Midland home. And when the Swansons visited Memphis, the Hayeses would return the favor when the two men played as partners in the fall classic at the Colonial Country Club, just a few blocks from Hayes's home.

When the guys were on the links, Colleen and Bea Hayes often would go shopping. Bea was a world-class shopper who enjoyed strolling the malls or inspecting the latest clothes on the rack. They'd pick up Christmas ornaments for their children and grandchildren. Other times, they would just curl up on a sofa together and talk. Bea had a great sense of humor and an effusive personality, and Colleen found her a welcome respite, someone who could easily take her mind off her troubles. Bea even shared Colleen's love for dogs, having taken one of the Swansons' Pug dog's offspring.

They were close enough friends, in fact, that whenever Hayes came through Midland, he would stop at the house, often without warning. They were good enough friends that Swanson would not have expected a call. So Hayes would surprise them, popping in unannounced as late as 9 P.M. for a quick visit and staying for dinner or drinks. The men could talk for hours, trading stories and gossip about mutual friends and colleagues at work.

Even though Hayes was the CEO of the subsidiary company, he remained an employee of Dow Corning Corporation. Because he was based in Memphis, Hayes often missed the scuttlebutt about who was ascending or descending the corporate ladder at headquarters in Midland. He relished every update Swanson could give him. And it was Dan and Bea who in late 1990 introduced John and Colleen to Sandestin, a residential beach resort located on the Gulf side of northwestern Florida. It is a little slice of paradise, replete with 64 holes of golf, where both couples acquired nearby condominiums.

Even their differing views of the breast implant crisis had failed to drive a wedge through their friendship. Long before the issue reached the front pages, Swanson and Hayes had engaged in several discussions about Dow Corning and implants. There was little overlap in their opinions. Hayes believed the company had become a victim of sensational media coverage and consumer politics. Swanson, of course, thought the company would come to regret its stonewalling tactics. For the sake of their friendship, however, they had both "agreed to disagree."

Now, with Dan and Bea planning a visit to Midland in early February 1992, Swanson planned to tell his friend the secret he had been carefully guarding for months—even if it cost him the friendship they had worked hard to maintain. When the Hayeses arrived at their home, Swanson opened a bottle of chardonnay and the two couples settled into the spacious living room that overlooked the Midland County Club golf course they had played on so many times together. Standing by the fireplace with glass in hand, he somehow summoned the courage to tell Hayes what he and Colleen had been awkwardly concealing for so long.

"There's something I've been wanting to tell you for a long time," Swanson said.

"Colleen had silicone implants...had many serious problems and last year had to have them removed."

He had expected Hayes to ask about his wife's health: Had she improved since the explantation? Hayes had long known of her bouts with fatigue, her frozen shoulder and her general malaise, and had never failed to inquire about how she was feeling during his past visits to the Swanson home.

Instead, Hayes said nothing. There was a long, awkward silence. He didn't know how to respond to this totally unexpected declaration.

"I know this implant mess has been hard on you, too," he said. "You've gone through hell, just as we have. Believe me, we've found lots of excuses not to tell you about Colleen. But we just didn't want you to hear it from anyone other than us. If it affects our friendship with you both, we will deeply regret it...but we will understand."

"I'm shocked," muttered Hayes. "I'm sorry to hear that."

Then, inexplicably, Hayes began a long, involved monologue about the future of silicone implants, the company's current position, and what the company would have to do to keep the devices on the market. It was as if a button had been pushed and Hayes had been programmed to give the company line and nothing more. He was already under intense pressure because of the crisis. The company was making Hayes ever more visible by attributing to him some of its most defensive and arrogant responses to each new piece of negative news. That put him directly in the media spotlight, in a public role he was not especially good at. Now, in this private moment with a friend, he was failing as well. Remarkably, Hayes showed little compassion for what the couple had been through, and no sympathy for Swanson's conflicted position in the company.

Meanwhile, Bea said nothing. Though rarely at a loss for words, she stared blankly at the floor in complete silence. The tension in the room was palpable.

Finally, Colleen asked Bea if she would like to go upstairs to see an old ice box that once belonged to her grandmother and had since been restored. "I didn't know how else to break the silence," recalls Colleen. "She seemed to be in absolute shock."

They left the men in the living room where Hayes continued to rattle on in a long, discomforting soliloquy. "Dan was on the defensive, under incredible pressure to defend the implants," recalls Swanson. "The pressure was enormous. He was going through the same kind of agony I was, but for totally different reasons. Dan will always be a good, loyal company person. In his case, I don't think you can separate the man from the organization. In fact, I'm not sure he could at that time separate his personal beliefs from those of the company's."

Colleen, meanwhile, said nothing more about her problems to Bea, and Bea didn't ask. When the women returned downstairs, Hayes had regained his composure. They had only stopped by to say hello, he said, and were on their way to dinner and then back to the Fairview Inn where they were staying. And with that, they quickly departed. When John and Colleen Swanson closed the door, they felt some relief—but much disappointment. Hayes had not expressed any concern about Colleen. He didn't even ask for any details about her condition.

Perhaps Hayes was embarrassed, humiliated, thought Swanson. On several occasions in the past, Colleen had bit her tongue as Hayes groused about "the crazy women" who were complaining about their implants. He often denounced the highly visible and vocal Sybil Goldrich, one of the founders of Command Trust Network, the group Colleen had turned to for help. Colleen had swallowed hard and let the comments pass without a word of judgment, seething inside. Hayes used to joke that he could immediately detect any woman with breast implants—no matter what she was wearing. But he apparently never knew Colleen had once had them.

The two couples made plans to have dinner a couple of nights later at one of the few places in Midland where one could get a good meal. That evening, at the Midland Country Club, breast implants were not discussed. Nor was Colleen's health. Indeed, Dan and Bea would never again ask about her health—until Bea herself became ill with cancer. "It was almost as if we never spoke to them about it," says Swanson. The four would see each other from time to time in the future. Swanson played his last invitational with Hayes that year, but their friendship would never again be the same.

The pressure on Hayes, as on every other executive involved in the crisis, continued to ratchet upward as critics continued to attack the company and its behavior. Hayes also became upset because the company decided in June 1992 to sell Dow Corning Wright and focus on its core businesses. The subsidiary, after all, had become a huge albatross. By the end of the year, Dow Corning would withdraw all silicone medical devices from the sales offering in an effort to protect itself from future litigation. The move, which would obviously affect the price Dow Corning would get for the business, was both a surprise and a personal setback for Hayes. By then, however, the company's senior executives just wanted out.

Although humor wasn't a staple within Dow Corning at the time, one enterprising member of the team assigned to help facilitate the sale of Dow Corning Wright brought some levity to the task in the form of a tongue-in-cheek board game. Called "Sell the Sucker!," the game was modeled after Monopoly. Written on the box that contained the game with its money in eight denominations, playing cards, and suited figures was: "Aspiring young executives can learn the rewards of good deeds and the consequences of naughty ones; the benefits of hard work and good decision-making and the harsh realities of slothfulness and poor decisions...played out against the backdrop of the rough-and-tumble corporate environment known as Dow Corning." One of the game's "Big Event" cards stated: "You notice that the Arlington Office Building has two offices with 'President' on the door. To cast your vote for Bob Rylee, stay on this space. To cast your vote

for Dan Hayes, move back one space. To cast your vote for
Bozo the Clown, move ahead one space."

Dow Corning finally rid itself of the subsidiary in May
1993, selling the assets of the company's large-joint orthopedic
device business for about $66 million to an investment part-
nership called Kidd Kamm Equity Partners in Greenwich,
Connecticut, and to Herbert W. Korthoff, a former executive of
United States Surgical Corporation. Rylee had put in a bid for
the business, but Dow Corning wasn't about to sell it to one of
its executives for fear of even more litigation down the road.

When Hayes finally retired from Dow Corning in 1993,
the Swansons listened as he made a rare admission before his
peers and his colleagues at a farewell party.

"I'm happy to be out of this," he said. "I'm totally burned
out."

*   *   *

Swanson wished he, too, could be out of it. Even though
he had officially removed himself from having anything to do
with breast implants, the issue wouldn't go away. It began to
take over the entire corporation. Simply booking one of the
conference rooms along the perimeter of the corporate center's hallways became increasingly difficult because they were
continually taken up by managers and employees dealing with
one aspect of the crisis or another—and no one wanted their
conversations overheard anymore. A general funk had come
over the corporate culture. Morale was falling. People were
distracted from the normal day-to-day business of the corporation.

Swanson couldn't even get his colleagues to honor his
recusal. Just before the FDA announced its moratorium on the
sale of silicone implants, he received a memo from Barbara
Carmichael, the communications vice-president, planning the
company's response to whatever action the agency might take.
Yet, Swanson had informed her in late September 1991 that a
"personal conflict of interest" prevented him from having any

involvement in the breast implant issue. "I reminded you of that on two occasions after the initial notification," wrote Swanson in a January 7, 1992, memo to Carmichael. "Now I am reminding you of it for the third time. If you need verification or confirmation, I advise you to speak with Kerm [Campbell]. You must somehow be convinced that I cannot be a part of this."

On the same day Swanson sent his agitated reply to Carmichael, he received an e-mail note from Robert Grupp, who was handling external communications on breast implants. Grupp asked him to prepare an official response for employees who were becoming upset about the huge amount of negative publicity the company was receiving on implants. "I know this is a 'drop everything' need...but that's been the nature of this corporate crisis," wrote Grupp. Swanson realized that Grupp had never been told of his recusal. "Bob," he wrote back, "I am not about to drop everything. Let's talk about this for a few minutes when you can." Little more than a month later, Swanson was invited to a meeting on Dow Corning's plans to cover and report on the FDA advisory panel meetings on implants.

Indeed, Swanson became increasingly frustrated by his company's inability to honor his request that he have nothing to do with implants. It was not that Campbell didn't agree with Swanson's position. Campbell, however, felt it was such a private matter that he hadn't shared Swanson's revelation with his colleagues. As a result, many of them weren't aware that Swanson was officially recused from the issue that was enveloping the entire corporation. He decided to seek out Dow Corning's new chairman and chief executive and inform him of his position.

Swanson had been in recusal for five months and wanted Keith McKennon to understand that he could not be counted upon for communications support on the implant issue. On the job for not much more than a week, McKennon had temporarily taken over Jack Ludington's old office on the third floor of DC-1. It was an open-plan office, surrounded by large, removable, curved sound-proofing barriers. Swanson had been in this office many times before because of his close association with Ludington over the years. Now his friend was gone and in his place was a tough, media savvy newcomer trying to get his hands around a monumental crisis.

Swanson had met McKennon on a few previous occasions because McKennon was chairman of the board committee that oversaw the company's ethics program. Every 18 months or so, Swanson was involved in a formal Business Conduct presentation to this audit and social responsibility committee. Swanson didn't know the executive well, but liked what he saw on the surface. McKennon was always pleasant and had displayed a good sense of humor. "Superficially, he's a hard person not to like," says Swanson.

For McKennon, it was a frenetic time. He was trying to get up to speed on the crisis as quickly as possible before departing for Washington and the FDA Advisory Panel sessions. He was scheduled to testify before the panel the next day, February 19. Swanson brought with him several memos, including the note he had written to his Business Conduct Committee colleagues after the *Business Week* story appeared in mid-1991.

McKeon welcomed Swanson into his office with a courteous, if perfunctory, handshake. If he didn't already know about Swanson's position—which he claimed he didn't—McKennon didn't seem surprised by it. He listened to what Swanson had to say about Colleen and his recusal. McKennon told Swanson he wanted to learn more about the issue and wanted to hear from women who had implants as well as scientists and doctors. He said he would be interested in chatting with Colleen upon his return from Washington, if possible, and Swanson said he would relay the request to his wife.

"I brought a few memos for you to read," Swanson said.

"Oh no," replied the always cautious McKennon, "I don't want those turning up in a lawsuit later on."

But McKennon accepted the information from Swanson, quickly digested the contents of the memos, and handed them back.

"What do you think Dow Corning's responsibility in this is?" asked McKennon.

The question caught Swanson off-guard.

"Keith," Swanson replied, "I haven't thought that through. I don't know what Dow Corning's responsibility is. I just wanted you to know I have a wife who is going through some very difficult times."

All told, the meeting lasted 15 to 20 minutes. When Swanson got back to his desk and jotted down a few notes on the session, he called the meeting a "sparring match." His sense was that McKennon was trying to size him up, find out whether he was sincere. Did he want to blackmail the company? What threat did he pose? Swanson, however, says he was motivated to approach McKennon out of fear that his wife's condition could be discovered and leaked. "The last thing we wanted to happen was to have her case publicly disclosed and inadvertently blindside Dow Corning," says Swanson. "Sharing my predicament with the company's CEO was in my view the ethical thing to do."

McKennon would get more bad news the day after testifying before the FDA. He had hoped to convince the agency, which had asked for the moratorium on their sale five weeks earlier, that silicone implants were safe. But the FDA advisory panel, after three hours of intense debate, voted to recommend that implants be taken off the market, with only a few exceptions for women requiring reconstruction after mastectomies or to correct serious deformities. All implant recipients would be required to enroll in clinical studies, and cosmetic augmentations would be limited to those in the clinical trials. FDA Commissioner Kessler had 60 days to rule on the panel's recommendation.

Two weeks later, on March 4, Swanson received a phone call from McKennon at his desk in the middle of the afternoon. McKennon was following up on his request to talk with Colleen. He maintained that he wanted to learn more about Colleen's problems. McKennon had already conducted dozens of media interviews, given a strong and compelling appearance on *Larry King Live,* and expressed what no other Dow Corning executive had ever dared say: that the company's overriding responsibility is to women with Dow Corning implants. While in Washington, McKennon had even had lunch with Sybil Goldrich of the Command Trust Network, who came to trust and like the executive. Unlike Reed, Rylee, Campbell, or Hayes, McKennon was listening to the other side and trying to appear compassionate without admitting there were any health or safety problems with the breast implants. At the FDA hearing, he said the company would "fully cooperate" with the FDA in its efforts to gather safety data on silicone implants.

On March 19, McKennon held a news conference at the National Press Club in Washington to announce that Dow Corning was quitting the breast implant business—regardless of what the FDA eventually decided. "It was my considered judgment that there was no viable market for these devices after all of this publicity and after these hearings, whether the commissioner raised the moratorium or not," said McKennon. "And I believed that Dow Corning had no viable business opportunity, pure and simple."

McKennon was now displaying visible leadership on this issue, something that had been lacking for several years. For his part, Swanson believed that the new CEO had begun to do some things that were long overdue. He had taken Dow Corning out of the breast implant business, established at least $10 million in funding for more research, provided up to $1200 each in financial help for women whose doctors recommended the removal of the implants, and just as important, displayed some compassion for women who suffered from illnesses attributed to their implants. "It was something, but too much damage had already been done," says Swanson. "Even the fireman couldn't turn back the clock."

Colleen, moreover, wasn't completely convinced of McKennon's motives. He was a public relations pro who had received plenty of ink for his success in defusing other controversies at Dow Chemical. The Swansons had already walked through the pros and cons of a meeting. Ultimately, however, it was Colleen's decision, and she didn't want to be part of what looked like a Dow Corning pacification program. Swanson told McKennon that Colleen had closely followed his trip to Washington and heard of his many meetings with other women who had problems with silicone implants.

"While she appreciates your interest," Swanson said, "Colleen doesn't think she could add much to your growing knowledge of silicone illnesses. Her problems aren't unique."

"That's unfortunate," McKennon said. "Look, I'll be glad to come out to your house, sit down in your living room."

But Swanson assured him that Colleen would not reconsider her decision. She simply could not see anything good coming from it. McKennon seemed disappointed by the answer, but accepted it graciously and hung up.

It was a rare day when Swanson didn't open up the *Midland Daily News* and see yet another story on breast implants, or turn on the television at home and see women who claimed to be Dow Corning victims. Even Dr. James Baker turned up on the *Phil Donohue Show,* on February 28, 1992, with his daughter Cindy, whom he had augmented with silicone implants at the age of 19. A stern Baker, sitting ramrod erect in a conservative suit with a white handkerchief tucked into his jacket breast pocket, criticized the FDA for its moratorium. "Anecdotal experience is not scientific fact," he said.

But on April 16, FDA Commissioner David Kessler concurred with the FDA advisory panel and banned silicone breast implants for most women because Dow Corning and the other manufacturers had not proven the devices were safe and effective. The 1976 Medical Device Amendment put the burden of proof that a product was safe and effective squarely on the manufacturer. Dow Corning and the other makers could not meet the burden to the FDA's satisfaction. Kessler noted that even though breast implants had been on the market for three decades, it still was not known how long the devices last or what percentage of them will rupture. Kessler said that studies on the basic characteristics of the product's performance such as tensile strength and fatigue resistance tested through cyclic loading were lacking. "The chemical composition of the gel that leaks into the body when a breast implant ruptures is unknown," said Kessler. "And the link, if any, between these implants and immune-related disorders and other systemic diseases is also unknown. Serious questions remain about the ability of the manufacturers to produce the device reliably and under strict quality controls."

The furor made Swanson decide to cancel a scheduled appearance in New York at the Conference Board's annual ethics program. How could he possibly address managers of other companies about ethics given his now awkward position at Dow Corning? Swanson began to notice that even his secretary of seven years, Maureen Pillepich, usually a sponge for gossip that she would readily use to entertain him and others, had become increasingly distant. She no longer freely volunteered information to her boss. And just before Kessler's controversial decision, Swanson was asked by General Counsel Jenkins to help the legal department deal with the management and ethical implications of breast implants. Despite his recusal, Swanson delivered a speech to some 40 corporate attorneys in a large conference room in DC-3. Without disclosing how the issue had affected him and his wife, he simply argued that Dow Corning should have quit the business on ethical grounds. He told the lawyers that all the scientific evidence to prove that silicone was unsafe still wasn't in, but the ethics of leaving the product on the market was another issue altogether. "They sat there like stones," recalls Swanson. No one challenged him. No one agreed with him, either.

When he traveled to Buenos Aires, Argentina, for a Business Conduct session that same month, Swanson found himself in a conference room surrounded by corrugated boxes stacked six feet high that were full of silicone breast implants. They were just some of the devices retrieved by Dow Corning's subsidiary in Argentina in the aftermath of the FDA's ban. Indeed, the country manager was having trouble getting all the implants returned from distributors who could still book a profit on them. Dow Corning was trying to do the right thing by taking them off the market entirely—even though they were not banned in Argentina—yet the company was having great difficulty convincing distributors to send them back. To the company's way of thinking, every silicone breast implant not retrieved represented a potential future lawsuit. Swanson felt as if he were in some *Twilight Zone* episode—he could not escape the issue, no matter where he went or what he did.

Sure enough, two months later, during a Business Conduct meeting in Wales, the plant manager of a Dow Corning facility in Barry showed him a tape of a recent BBC television program on silicone breast implants that opened with a huge ball exploding into an orange inferno. It was a film clip of napalm made by Dow Chemical. Breast implants, the announcer sarcastically reported, came from the same people who brought the public napalm.

*　　*　　*

As the pressure on the company grew, Swanson felt the heavy weight of it on himself as well. During the day, his stomach would heave with pain. He consumed Maalox like it was water, but the upset would never really go away. His back began to trouble him as well. Swanson's doctor told him that stress was a great part of it. He said that the stress on the company from all the media coverage on breast implants must have taken a toll on Swanson. Little did the doctor know, thought Swanson, that the media attention was something of a relief. "The emotion was inside and it was churning," he recalls. "The harder I tried to keep up the appearances, the more it affected me internally. I was always tired. My back was giving me fits. I wasn't digesting food properly. My stomach always hurt. It was hard to put on a good face to go to work, and yet I had to do this. I did not want to appear negative or arrogant or belligerent or adversarial to the company. I worked very hard to maintain a good demeanor, but it wasn't easy. Anybody in a corporate setting and in recusal for a time is going to have problems. The stress is just there and you can't avoid it unless you're totally devoid of feelings." His nights became increasingly restless. At one point, he went to a sleep clinic in Saginaw, where he was told, among other things, to avoid caffeine and use a different pillow. None of it helped. There were nights when he failed to get even an hour's sleep.

He thought of quitting his job altogether. But Colleen's medical bills averaged $50,000 to $60,000 a year from 1991 to 1993, making it impossible for him to walk out and away from his medical coverage and future retirement benefits. Swanson prayed that he could hang on for just a little more time, because he had already notified the company of his intention to retire as soon as he was eligible to do so—in August 1993.

Moreover, he had no way of knowing how long Colleen would be ill or what disaster was waiting around the next corner. Even though her implants were out, she was not doing well. She had lost so much weight that one neighbor asked if she was anorexic. She was frail. Her general health was not good. She had begun to lose her hair. There were periodic rashes on her upper body and chest. She had developed a condition called Raynaud's disease, causing a white discoloration of her skin on some extremities. "For us, it was sort of like we were in an incubator and couldn't get out," he says. "We were trapped there. We knew that there would be an end point, but I don't know how we would have felt if I had ten years more to work. What kept me going was my belief that my position was correct and the corporation was wrong. If I had been on the line and vacillated, it would have been devastating."

To ease his tension, Swanson would take long walks on the 120 acres of the Midland County Club's golf course. He would take their dog, a Pug named Joy, and circle the course early in the mornings or in the evenings after dinner. On his strolls, he would sometimes think back to his days as a teenager in Minneapolis, when he began to caddie. His father and many of the men in his family had played the game. And, of course, he would wonder how all of it would end.

His walks, lasting 45 minutes or so, would usually take Swanson to the north end of the clubhouse near the sixth hole, not far from the Alden Dow–designed home of Dow Corning President Larry Reed. He rarely saw Reed on the course since Reed avoided club-sponsored golf events, preferring to play by himself or, occasionally, in the early evening hours with his wife, Lois Ann. Swanson had, however, had at least one opportunity to play golf with Reed, in the summer of 1989, when Reed had called him at work and asked him to play that afternoon. Reed had been anxious to squeeze in some practice just before heading out to New York to play in the Pro-Am event at the annual Corning Classic tournament. Swanson, however, had been truly bogged down, had a previously scheduled evening engagement, and so had done the politically incorrect thing: He turned down the chance to walk the links with Dow Corning's chief executive and president. "It wasn't a very smart thing to do," admits Swanson, "and I probably would have enjoyed it, but I was up against some tough deadlines."

Late in 1990, the Swansons joined St. John's Episcopal Church, located not far from their home, and the two ministers there provided great comfort to Colleen, especially after her implants were removed. Still, neither Swanson nor his wife felt they could speak openly about their problems because the community was so small and enclosing. "All we really had was each other," says Swanson. "We didn't have *many* other outlets." Colleen confided in her daughter, Kathy, but Swanson had no place to turn. Besides Hayes, another of his closest friends was Larry Kotter, then Dow Corning's director of corporate purchasing: Swanson felt that Kotter, like Hayes, would probably not be sympathetic to his belief that the company had been involved in anything wrong or unethical. He was exactly what Swanson had been, a company man.

Even his daily walks across the manicured greens of the golf course would soon be taken from him. The Swansons sold their lovely home in September 1992, because Colleen could no longer negotiate the steep stairs and in anticipation of a slump in Midland's real estate market. The Dow Chemical Company, like many other large, over-staffed U.S. companies, was preparing to downsize its operations and reduce costs. Swanson knew that any sizable layoff would quickly depress the town's real estate market, which was heavily affected by Dow's personnel decisions. So the couple put their house up for sale, sold it quickly, and moved into a condominium just a block away from Dow Chemical's corporate headquarters. It was a pleasant, if dull, neighborhood, largely composed of very young singles and retired people. It was nothing like the home and environment they had given up on the golf course.

*   *   *

With Colleen Swanson's health problems only worsening, she finally decided to sue her husband's employer. To be sure, she and John Swanson had talked it through thoroughly. "It's not going to make things any easier for me at Dow Corning," Swanson had said. At the same time, he knew that Colleen had every right to sue his employer for the damage she believed her silicone implants had caused. He would not be a party to the lawsuit. He could not, in fact, have any communication with her attorney during the duration of the litigation.

Dow Corning's legal department had been informed of a possible suit from Colleen in January 1991 by a Chicago attorney, Ken Moll, who Colleen had been referred to by the Command Trust. Moll suggested to Dow Corning that he come to Midland and speak with the company's attorneys about a settlement that might avoid a lawsuit. Greg Thiess, the same attorney who had earlier delivered Rylee's message to Dillon, said Dow Corning had no interest in such a meeting and left it at that.

At that time, Colleen was still without medical documentation that her illness was definitely caused by silicone. Dr. Richard Stein, a Cleveland rheumatologist who worked closely with Dr. Feng, had examined her on January 6, 1992. His diagnosis: "With her Raynaud's, fatigue, arthralgias, and chest wall pain it appears she probably does, in fact, have a silicone-related disease. Whether this represents human adjuvant disease or not, I cannot state for certain." Dr. Feng had referred Colleen to yet another Cleveland doctor, gynecologist Henry Yarboro, who performed a D and C on Colleen in February because her periods had become erratic, with excessive bleeding and bloodclotting. A month after performing the procedure, Yarboro told Colleen that a hysterectomy would probably be necessary.

Another examination by Dr. Stein on July 17, 1992, led to a more definitive diagnosis. "At this point," Stein wrote in his medical records, "after a year's worth of experience in dealing with well over 100 women with silicone implants, it is my opinion that she, in fact, does have a silicone associated disease. Her prognosis is quite guarded at this time, as most women do not seem to respond to removal of the implants...."

With this diagnosis in hand, Colleen finally decided to file suit against Dow Corning. Her first attorney, Ken Moll, was not licensed to practice in Michigan, where the suit would be filed, so he referred her to a local lawyer, Mark A. Kolka of Allsopp, Kolka and Wackerly in nearby Bay City, Michigan. The last thing she wanted, however, was to see a headline in a newspaper about the spouse of a Dow Corning executive filing a lawsuit. So she insisted that the papers be filed late on a Friday afternoon, just minutes before the Michigan state court in Bay City closed its doors, to minimize the chance that a reporter would discover the documents and write a story on them. The suit was filed on August 21, 1992.

Kolka, whose father had been a chemical engineer for Dow Chemical, had handled the usual array of auto negligence, worker safety, product liability, and medical malpractice cases. He had become interested in breast implants after a friend of his daughter visited with him in 1987. The woman, Alison Cardinal, who was 24 years old, had a single implant in her left breast because the breast had failed to develop. She had been implanted at the age of 15. Subsequently, the implant had ruptured. It rolled up and sat on her shoulder when she lay down. When the surgeons tried putting another one in, the incision failed to heal properly.

To Kolka, it was a straight product liability case. He had discovered through his contacts with other trial attorneys that Dow Corning was typically settling rupture cases out of court for not much more than $30,000 each. After speaking with attorney Dan Bolton in San Francisco, however, Kolka began to examine, as part of the discovery process for the Cardinal case, hundreds of thousands of documents at Dow Corning's medical plant in Hemlock. "It was gold," he says. "I was surprised and offended by what I saw. It was amazing that they hadn't burned or destroyed them."

When he pressed the Cardinal suit, what amazed him was how hard Dow Corning fought back. "They did everything they could to delay, to hinder discovery, to omit facts, to disguise the truth," claims Kolka, who can scarcely disguise his dislike for the company or its executives. "They are masters of omission. They just pissed me off with their tactics." At one point, for example, Dow Corning refused to certify that the documents Kolka had photocopied from the company's own files were authentic—an issue that the two sides contested all the way to the Michigan Court of Appeals, where Dow Corning claimed it would cost more than $100,000 simply to verify the authenticity of the documents. The court rejected the argument, refusing to overrule a trial judge. Eventually, Kolka won an undisclosed settlement for Cardinal and picked up more than a dozen other breast implant cases along with Colleen's.

*   *   *

In the spirit of open communications, Chairman and CEO McKennon agreed to periodically provide employees with updates about the ongoing breast implant crisis. On November 4, 1992, in the basement cafeteria of the corporate center in DC-1, Swanson listened to McKennon discuss the recent completion of Griffin Bell's investigation. Bell's law firm of King and Spalding had been hired in January, before McKennon came to Dow Corning.

On this day, McKennon told some 200 assembled employees that Bell's team had interviewed 250 people and collected 300,000 documents during their nine-month probe. "Employees should feel good about the Bell investigation results," he said. The recommendations by Bell, McKennon emphasized, did not raise any significant new public health issues.

The recommendations from Bell's law firm, which reputedly had been billing Dow Corning as much as $1 million a month for its services, were fairly innocuous. They urged the company to make all nonprivileged documents reviewed by King and Spalding available to the FDA along with a list of all the witnesses interviewed by the law firm.

The only negative finding—and the only one to make headlines—was the conclusion that Dow Corning employees had, over the years, falsified manufacturing records for several batches of silicone implants. Some employees doctored records of the oven temperatures at which liquid silicone had been heated before being placed in the implant envelopes. The heating process turned liquid silicone into a thick gel, making it less likely to ooze from the implant.

Although the company became aware of the problem in 1987 and had disciplined the employees involved, few outside Dow Corning had known about the incident, which raised still more questions about the company's quality control. Critics maintained that such deviations in the manufacturing process meant the silicone in the implants wasn't of uniform consistency or chemical content and increased the likelihood of gel bleed—an issue that had come up in some court cases where the problem had already surfaced but had been kept under wraps by Dow Corning through protective court orders. McKennon, however, told reporters that he was "satisfied there weren't cases where there was insufficient time and temperature" to cook the gel.

While this was news to Swanson, it was hardly of major import. What surprised him was McKennon's disclosure that the company would not make public the final report of the Bell team but only its rather mild recommendations. McKennon said the undisclosed part of the report would, in fact, be used in the company's legal defense. To Swanson, it was a significant disappointment that the supposedly objective investigation would now be used to defend the company's behavior. Swanson believed that decision represented a conflict of interest on the part of both Dow Corning and the law firm. How could King and Spalding legitimately investigate the company's behavior, yet also gather information for Dow Corning to use against plaintiffs in courtrooms?

Swanson mentioned his concerns about McKennon's comments to Jan Botz, a protégé who had assumed a part of his communication responsibilities after his recusal. She was noncommittal, but quickly relayed Swanson's concerns to McKennon, who called later in the afternoon and asked that he drop by his office for a few minutes. McKennon didn't mention the subject of the meeting, and Swanson didn't bother to ask. He knew why McKennon wanted to see him.

"By that point in time, my position had been pretty well consolidated in my own thinking and I was living with it," Swanson recalls. "I felt that I was right in this whole issue. If you hire an outside law firm to investigate your conduct and give the firm full and free access to look into all your affairs, you're ostensibly doing it to gain credibility with your constituencies inside and outside the company. That's what I felt was the sole purpose of the undertaking. Now to hear in the employee forum that there was another agenda, another reason for commissioning the Bell investigation, raised a question in my mind. I wanted [McKennon] to know that at least one person in the audience had a concern about it."

Swanson found McKennon sitting behind the conference table in his office. The CEO told Swanson that Botz had said Swanson was troubled by McKennon's announcement at the forum. Swanson replied that some would interpret the decision to use the findings in defense of the company as an ethical breach.

"How could Bell do an objective investigation of Dow Corning and also help the company prepare its legal defense?" asked Swanson. "I wouldn't be surprised if the company received more criticism from the media if the existence of this hidden report became widely known."

McKennon immediately became defensive. "I can look you right in the eye and tell you that there was never any intent to do anything unethical or underhanded," McKennon insisted. "I swear to you, there was no hidden agenda. There was no ethical violation here."

The meeting broke up within 5 or 10 minutes. But the two would meet again five days later, when McKennon finally was told of Colleen's lawsuit. Much to Swanson's amazement, Dow Corning's legal department had not informed McKennon of the lawsuit until nearly three months after it was filed. Realiz-ing the implications of the case, McKennon called Swanson on November 9 and asked him to come to his office yet again.

When Swanson arrived only a few minutes later, McKennon seemed tense and ill at ease. He told Swanson he had heard about Colleen's lawsuit within the past few days and wished that he had known about it earlier. Swanson listened as he vent-ed his frustrations. In this situation, he did not appear any-where near as smooth and confident as he had when he had faced Larry King on live television. McKennon told him there had been no need for a lawsuit, that the company could have handled the problem another way. Swanson explained that a month before McKennon joined Dow Corning, Colleen's origi-nal attorney in Chicago, Ken Moll, had called Thiess to propose coming to Midland to work out a resolution and avoid a lawsuit. But Dow Corning's attorneys had denied the request and insist-ed that Colleen's case be handled like any other. McKennon was clearly upset by the news. He obviously knew the company faced another public relations disaster if word got out that the wife of a Dow Corning executive had sued the company over silicone breast implants. "I had never seen him this angry," recalls Swanson. "He was mad, first at me, and then, I suppose, at the legal department."

"Look," a red-faced McKennon demanded loudly, "What does Colleen want out of this? Does she want a zillion dollars? This could be messy. Can't we just talk this out and see if we can get it resolved?"

The more Swanson and McKennon spoke about the law-suit, however, the more it became apparent that they were resolving nothing. Finally, McKennon suggested that perhaps he and Colleen could sit down and talk about the case away from Dow Corning. His only purpose in meeting Colleen would be to avoid what McKennon said "could be a messy situation." Once again, Swanson agreed to play the role of the intermediary, take it up with his wife, and get back to him as soon as possible.

Before Swanson left the office, though, McKennon asked what he would do after he retired from Dow Corning. Swanson told him he planned to remain active in the field of business ethics, possibly as a consultant, and that there was a real possibility that he would do some writing on ethics.

"Would you be writing about Dow Corning?" asked McKennon.

"Very possibly," answered Swanson. "It's an interesting case."

"Oh," the CEO said, with a frown. "I sure do respect your views and your right to express them. But y'know, John, you've got to be careful."

Three days later, on November 12, the two men were facing each other again. Swanson had initiated a follow-up meeting to tell McKennon that Colleen had thought about his offer and decided that she would speak to him only with her attorney present. She had asked Kolka for his opinion and he had ad-vised her that it would be a bad idea to meet alone with the chairman of Dow Corning about her suit.

"Look," Swanson said, "I can't undo this. Colleen can't undo this. This was filed months ago. If our legal department had been willing to talk to Colleen when her attorney called the first time in 1991, I probably wouldn't be here talking to you about this today. But that obviously didn't happen, and now it's flowing through the legal process. Keith, I doubt very much if Colleen would talk to you now, one on one, about her case without legal representation. It's simply gone too far."

McKennon said that wasn't what he had in mind. He was doubtful that a meeting with lawyers present would be very productive. Still, McKennon said he would speak to the legal department about it.

"I wish we could have worked this out another way," McKennon said, ending the meeting. "It looks like this will be messy." It was the last time Swanson and McKennon would meet.

A FINAL
ASSIGNMENT

For Dow Corning Corporation, the mess only grew messier. Under pressure from Congress, the FDA publicly requested the full Bell report from Dow Corning. (Ultimately, Dow Corning fought the request in court and won. Led by Sidney Wolfe, Public Citizen on January 14, 1993 called for criminal charges to be brought against Dow Corning. The next month, the Department of Justice subpoenaed the company in an investigation to determine whether Dow Corning had misled doctors and their patients about the safety of silicone implants. A grand jury was convened in Baltimore to investigate the charges, which were later dismissed. And so many women filed lawsuits against the company—more than 15,000—that Dow Corning eventually began to explore the possibility of putting together what would become the largest product liability pact in history. The $4.3 billion agreement would offer compensation to any woman in the world with illnesses allegedly linked to silicone breast implants.

Even though the controversy raged on, by January 1993 Keith McKennon had signaled his intent to relinquish his responsibilities as chief executive of Dow Corning by the end of the year. By being open and more visible, McKennon had at least kept the company afloat through the crisis. And there was no doubt that he was fully in charge. Richard A. Hazleton, an unassuming and little-known chemical engineer who was then running Dow Corning's European operations, was called back to become president and McKennon's heir-apparent.

Swanson, already counting the days to an early retirement

that would allow him to escape from Dow Corning and Midland, was delighted by the news. When he first moved to Midland, Hazleton had been his next-door neighbor on Salem Street. A Chicago native, Hazleton had joined the company in 1965 after graduating from Purdue University—just a year before Swanson moved to Midland. Hazleton was not a flashy or high-profile executive. He looked like any of the many engineers who so often climbed Dow Corning's corporate ladder: He wore glasses and was partial to short-sleeved shirts. He didn't mind that pens stuck out from his shirt pocket. He preferred anonymity to public visibility.

Swanson had watched as Hazleton migrated from a series of engineering jobs into finance until 1983 when the executive made a major leap in his career, taking control of Dow Corning's huge Midland factory. Swanson became reacquainted with his old neighbor when Hazleton served on the corporate Business Conduct Committee from 1987 to 1990. Then Hazleton was sent to Europe to streamline the company's operations. Though Swanson had been disturbed when Hazleton asked him not to attend the meeting to resolve the Dillon conflict, Swanson thought Hazleton was a reasonable choice to lead Dow Corning into the future. He respected the man's values and judgments. Soon after the announcement of Hazleton's promotion, Swanson sent him a memo on business ethics that would lead to one last assignment before Swanson retired from the company.

Discussing the failure of the ethics program to prevent the silicone implant crisis, Swanson wrote:

> Does that mean that our past business conduct practices were wrong or a waste of time and energy? No. We have built up a reservoir of good will among employees and...among our key customers.

> What I think it does mean is that how Dow Corning is being perceived by the media, government, the regulatory agencies, courts and special interest groups should tell us that the standards we've used in the past to judge our conduct are out of touch with the world we live in. I think of our business conduct processes as "Good Time Ethics"...appro-

priate for the long-gone time when Dow Corning was…insu-
lated from and immune to the slings and arrows suffered by
the Exxons, Union Carbides, and Merrill Lynches of the
world. I also believe that if we look deeply into our past
ethics processes, we would have to reluctantly conclude that
they have not been closely enough connected to anything
that's really important to the corporation. (And it hurts to
say that.)

Hazleton did not share Swanson's belief that the breast
implant controversy was an ethical dilemma for the company.
For him, it was a business problem. Nonetheless, Hazleton,
then 50, suggested that Swanson devote his last few months
at the company to ethics alone. Swanson's final job was to
assess, evaluate, and critique the business conduct process
that he had guided for nearly 17 years.

Swanson sometimes wondered if he had been given the
assignment because it was important to Dow Corning or
because the company feared that he and Colleen might appear
on some TV talk show, only to stir up more controversy and
trouble. The company already was concerned that Swanson
might write a book on his experiences. Whatever the reason, it
was clear that he was slowly coming to be seen as an outsider
on the inside. McKennon, who would have considered the
possibility of a book by Swanson an act of treason, asked his
staffers to more thoroughly question Swanson about his intentions. On November 24, for example, in-house attorney John
Rigas privately met with Swanson in a DC-2 conference room.
During the meeting, Rigas gently probed Swanson's plans with
a lawyer-like demeanor. At one point, recalls Swanson, he suggested that Dow Corning and Swanson consider a collaboration on a book project.

The thought seemd preposterous to John Swanson. "It
wouldn't make any sense," he told Rigas. "My point of view is
dramatically different from the corporation's, and I can't see
how any oversight from our legal department would lend itself
to a credible book." Rigas listened closely, displaying no emotion or reaction to the remarks that Swanson knew would be
promptly relayed to Keith McKennon. Shortly after his session

with Rigas, Swanson was no longer allowed to attend the company's monthly management communication meetings.

In March 1993, Swanson moved out of his communications office and onto the third floor of DC-1 to report directly to Hazleton. He moved from a cramped beehive of corporate activity to more spacious and hushed quarters on the floor where the senior corporate executives had their offices. But Swanson's new professional home was in the auditing department, on the opposite side of the building from Hazleton and the other top executives. It had the quiet, well-ordered feel of a study area in a library.

For Swanson, there was isolation and solitude. "There was no action, no noise, nothing," he recalls. "This was the final stage of recusal. It was the last stop on the train, and from here I would depart. But I was determined to be productive. I was not going to spend eight months looking out a window." Swanson did work hard, but not at the often frenetic pace he had been accustomed to. There was little, if any, pressure on him to perform. There were no regular deadlines he had to meet. There were few colleagues, other than a handful on the Business Conduct Committee, with whom he interacted.

*   *   *

Besides coming up with a sheaf of recommendations for forging a better ethics program, Swanson had to cope with the other pressures that had been weighing on him for months. Colleen was not getting any better despite the explantation. He had to move out of Midland and find a new place to live. And he had to put everything that had happened behind him. "Colleen was constantly sick," he says. "My job was a problem. We tended to shy away from people who talked about implants and started to socialize with friends who had nothing to do with Dow Corning. We made some serious sacrifices in our own quality of life in order not to involve people in our concerns and attitudes when they held different opinions. As good as most people were at Dow Corning about it, there was still a stigma. It sets you aside. It's not as if you have leprosy, but you are different."

That difference was real and palpable. Rumors about the Swansons were spreading throughout the community. It wasn't possible to keep a lid on them. Swanson, for example, heard that the wife of a Dow Corning executive had been gossiping about Colleen and her lawsuit at a retiree board meeting in July. Trying to trace the source, Swanson called her up and asked where she heard about it. She told him the story had come from another executive's wife, whose husband had picked it up at a meeting of Dow Corning managers.

Colleen's final year in Midland was a horrendous one. In March 1993, she returned to Cleveland for a hysterectomy and the removal of her ovaries by Dr. Henry Yarboro, who had been recommended by Dr. Lu-Jean Feng. Shortly after returning to Midland, however, Colleen found that her urine was draining through her vagina. She went back to Cleveland to yet another doctor, Sidney Cohen, chief of urology at Mount Sinai Hospital, who detected a hole in her bladder and inserted a catheter to drain her urine. For several days, Colleen suffered nausea, cramps, diarrhea, and loss of appetite.

Finally, on the morning of March 28, she entered the Midland Hospital emergency room with severe shakes and nausea. Since the explantation, all of her medical needs related in any way to problems caused by silicone implants had been taken care of outside of Midland. Now, John was taking her to a Midland hospital, where they would have to disclose that Colleen Swanson, the wife of a Dow Corning executive, had once had silicone implants and had been diagnosed with silicone-related disease. Two members of the hospital's board of trustees were Dow Corning executives. Several nurses at the hospital were married to Dow Corning employees. "We had no choice but to disclose the information," says Swanson. "But we had to assume it probably would filter out. That bothered us greatly because we had worked so hard for so long to keep this contained. Now there was the real possibility that it would blow up."

The hospital staff irrigated Colleen's bladder and checked

her out of the emergency room. She returned to the hospital by ambulance later that night when her shakes became so extreme that Swanson thought his wife was going to die. Colleen was now so weak that John could not carry her into his car as he had earlier in the day. So he followed the ambulance, its siren wailing, to the hospital. He watched through the back windows of the van as the medical technicians struggled to keep Colleen conscious by asking her to count backwards and name past presidents. Her vital signs and white blood count were abnormal, and she was admitted by Dr. Tammy Phillips, who started heavy antibiotics and intravenous feeding.

When the doctor ordered a CAT scan to check for the possibility of blood clots in her lungs, Colleen suffered a severe allergic reaction to the dyes injected into her for the procedure. Her blood pressure shot up, and she experienced chest pains and difficulty breathing. As she lay on the table in pain, the hospital staffers were yelling over her body to notify her husband because she was so close to death.

Fortunately, Colleen pulled through. On April 3, 1993, she was released from the hospital, only to return three days later for surgery to repair the hole in her bladder. Colleen, however, continued to feel nauseated and lacked much of an appetite, causing her to lose still more weight and suffer from dehydration. She was sent back to Midland Hospital's emergency room to be fed intravenously and to be given medicines to alleviate the severe nausea. For a time nothing seemed to work. Her weight fell to a mere 89 pounds from a normal weight of 104. It would be months before she began a slow recovery that would continue after her husband retired from Dow Corning and she left Midland.

Yet, through all her ups and downs, Colleen had to acknowledge that the decision to have implants in the first place had been hers. She had been assured by perhaps the most knowledgeable source that the devices were safe, that the operation was riskfree, and that the implants would last a lifetime—all false or exaggerated promises. But the decision to have cosmetic surgery had been hers alone. It was a decision that continued to cause her pain, to nag at her just as consistently as the pain she felt in her joints, the migraines, and the extreme fatigue that proved so debilitating. It was a decision that she still kept secret, refusing to inform even her parents that she had had implants and they were the cause of her health problems. Colleen could not yet admit to them that she had undergone unnecessary surgery to make herself look better. "I should have been secure enough in my own mind to accept myself just the way I was," she says now. "If John was willing to accept me, why did I have to change it? It was a very stupid thing to do. It's something I will regret for the rest of my life."

                    *   *   *

As Swanson performed his final corporate task, he reviewed the entire crisis. He became convinced that there were numerous decisions made by the company and its executives that had been the wrong ones. Dow Corning, Swanson thought, made a mistake in the mid-1960s when it decided to enter the business without, in his opinion, adequately testing silicone breast implants. And it made a mistake again in 1976, when it decided to stay in the business after Congress granted the FDA authority to regulate medical devices. Dow Corning, Swanson thought, should have re-assessed the future of its implant business in light of the cost of safety studies the FDA would soon require. Instead, Swanson believed, the company rushed to market a new, thin-shelled breast implant.

In 1978, when Swanson had made sure that a challenging question was asked of the company's executives at the media training session, the impact had been negligible. The question alone, and the *Ms.* magazine article that prompted it, should have led the executives to question why the company was in the breast implant business and then investigate the consequences of staying in the business.

An even more obvious time for management to reexamine the business had come in 1984, when Dow Corning lost the Maria Stern lawsuit, the first court case in which the company was accused of fraud and negligence. Instead of deciding that the jury's verdict was "an aberration," Swanson thought, the company should have dug more deeply into the reasons for the loss. Management, he believed, should have looked more closely at the damaging documents unearthed for the trial from Dow Corning's own files.

Three years later, an internal group had conducted what had been known as the "gel tox review" to study concerns that silicone could cause cancer. Although the review had laid those concerns to rest, the company had discovered that it had no studies of any consequence on auto-immune problems. Swanson thought the company could simply have decided then whether it wanted to spend several million dollars on such studies or make the decision that this was a business it should no longer be in. And a year later, in 1988, when the FDA put the company on notice that within three years it would have to prove the safety and effectiveness of the devices, Swanson thought Dow Corning had had still another opportunity either to pull out of the market or to fund the long-term clinical studies it did not have.

There had been more warning signals. In 1989, the FDA had reclassified silicone breast implants as potentially carcinogenic. In 1990, the National Center for Health Statistics had published the results of a survey showing far higher rupture, complication, and removal rates for silicone implants than those stated by Dow Corning. Then, in mid-1991, there had been *Business Week's* allegations that Dow Corning had known for a decade or more that silicones could cause health problems.

Ultimately, though, Swanson concluded that the company's troubles with breast implants had been preordained by its sheltered corporate upbringing, the homogeneity of its work force, and a consummate and arrogant belief in its own scientific superiority. Protected from public scrutiny and accountable only to its two shareholders—Dow Chemical and Corning Incorporated—the company had grown up without having to face the rigors that beset publicly owned corporations.

When serious questions about the safety of silicones began turning up on the evening news in 1990 thanks to consumer advocates like Sydney Wolfe, Sybil Goldrich, and Kathleen Anneken, Dow Corning's management had been shocked and bewildered. The company, thought Swanson, had gone into a state of denial. As well it might. In the Dow Corning culture, science and technology reigned supreme. When he first joined the company, one of the very first things he had learned about silicone was that it did not react with anything, least of all the human body. But years later, in August 1992, the British medical journal *Lancet* had published the results of a study indicating that silicones can create antibodies in human beings. Subsequent stories in the business press had been laden with comments from credible scientists who discussed linkages between silicone gel implants and a number of never-before-seen diseases of the human immune system. And even Dow Corning, in March 1993, had acknowledged for the first time that silicone may not be inert after all. The company had publicly conceded that one of its own studies on laboratory rats had found a possible link between silicone implants and auto-immune system irregularities. "It clearly raises my concern that silicone gel might cause immune-system disease," Dr. Myron Harrison, Dow Corning's chief medical officer, was quoted as saying.

Swanson's fields were communications and business ethics; he was not a chemist or a scientist. He couldn't argue the merits of the scientific debate. And conflicting evidence would later emerge about the safety of implants. A University of Michigan study, funded by Dow Corning, would find no link between implants and the immune-system disease sclero-derma. Another study by the Mayo Clinic, partly funded by Dow Corning through contributions to plastic surgeons, would supposedly find no connection between breast implants and connective-tissue diseases. But each of these studies, which seemed to support Dow Corning's position, would be quickly attacked by critics who faulted the research methodology.

Swanson didn't know who was right, and he still doesn't. He is certain, in fact, that all the scientific proof is not yet in. But he has no doubt that Dow Corning behaved unethically.

The company failed to provide the women who decided to have implants the opportunity to give their informed consent. For years, women had not been fully aware of the risks they were incurring to have Dow Corning silicone in their bodies. And only after losing a major court battle had the company begun to change the inserts that were included in the implant packages to more fully disclose the risks. The company had failed to act quickly on the numerous complaints it received from its own sales staff and from plastic surgeons who bought its products. The company had failed to promptly do the follow-up testing its own scientists had been urging it to do for years.

In Swanson's view, Dow Corning's elaborate ethics program failed the breast implant test because of what he perceived to be an unresolved conflict in the organization between moral behavior and profits. When several scientists had urged more research on potential problems such as those that afflicted Colleen, the company's management had hesitated to fund the necessary studies. They were, after all, highly expensive studies on a relatively minor product that was making little, if any, money for the company. The cost-benefit analysis didn't seem to work in favor of extensive safety testing on a product the company had sold for nearly 30 years.

Swanson believed the company had failed to live up to its own code of conduct on at least two major points. The code pledged that the company would "be responsible for the impact of Dow Corning's technology upon the environment." In Swanson's judgment, the company had failed that standard when it claimed that ultimate responsibility lay with its direct customer—plastic surgeons.

The code also stated that Dow Corning would "continually strive to assure that our products and services are safe, efficacious and accurately represented in our selling and promotional activities." Here too, in Swanson's view, the company had failed to meet its own ethical standards. Dow Corning's senior management, of course, did not believe the breast implant issue was an ethical problem. And despite his suggestions to the contrary, Swanson and the Business Conduct Committee had not been asked to get involved.

Instead, short-term survival strategies urged on the company's leadership by lawyers had won out over "doing the right thing." At the peak of the controversy, the company had lacked a strong, morally motivated leader, thought Swanson. "Dow Corning's handling of the implant crisis proved that the best of ethics programs can't be effective in a serious crisis unless they are visibly supported at the top," insists Swanson. That support had been sorely lacking when Chief Executive Larry Reed, who was supposed to be in charge of the controversy, had delegated the problem to a lieutenant and kept a low profile. Instead of using the company's code of conduct as a guide to help manage the crisis, Reed had adopted a defensive, almost arrogant, position, expressing no empathy, at least publicly, for the thousands of women who complained that Dow Corning's implants caused them pain and suffering.

In the end, thought Swanson, it mattered little whether the company's executives truly believed that its implants were safe or not. "The issue for me had little to do with the current status of silicone science. As far as I was concerned, the definitive answers were still in the future. The here-and-now issue for me was the company's callousness, its insensitivity, and its unwillingness to acknowledge that there were women who truly believed that their implants were the root cause of the health problems. I had failed to convince Dow Corning's top management that the implant controversy was not just a matter of what science was right and what science was wrong. At the height of the public controversy in 1991 and 1992, it really didn't matter, since there were no clear answers about the science of silicones. But there was a rapidly growing body of anecdotal evidence that reasonable people could not ignore."

Most of all, Swanson learned much about himself. Like many managers, he had faced difficult problems over the years, from budget crunches to personnel cutbacks. Unlike most managers, however, he had also worked through hundreds of thorny ethical issues as part of his business conduct responsibilities. Through those years, four pillars of ethical conduct had served him well: honesty, fairness, keeping commitments, and respecting the dignity of the individual. He had always tried his best to observe these guidelines himself and continually stressed their importance in the hundreds of business conduct reviews he had led over 18 years. But for Swanson, the breast implant controversy—in which the company's integrity was pitted against his own conclusions about the dangers of silicone implants and the company's long-time knowledge of them—was like no other ethical dilemma he had dealt with.

In his final days at the company, Swanson came to realize and accept that sometimes you have to face a deep and burdensome crisis alone, that sometimes you have to put your career and your financial obligations to one side. He learned that no matter how well intentioned a corporate ethics program might be, it would not work if it was ignored in a crisis. "There are no pat processes or tried-and-true mechanisms to resolve these isolated and rare predicaments," he says. "In my case, there was no one inside the company to whom I could turn for counsel. I had no way of knowing for sure where the loyalties of even my closest Dow Corning colleagues and friends would be. But I had to believe that when push came to shove, very few of my colleagues would be willing to put their own careers on the line for the sake of an ethical concern that one person thought was important."

In an increasingly tenuous corporate world, ever fewer people may sacrifice their careers for some moral or ethical issue. But Swanson came to believe that something he called "the sovereignty of the spirit" was far more important than success. He meant by that the yearning to do what he believed to be the right thing, despite any fallout that might result. "I had become convinced beyond a doubt that Dow Corning had not been honest or fair with a million or so women with silicone breast implants," Swanson says. "The company had not lived up to its commitments as expressed in the code of conduct. The company had also violated the dignity of many of those women who had placed their unsuspecting trust in a manufacturer's claim that the implants were safe. What I am less sure of is how much of my ultimate conviction could be attributed to my close and very personal involvement in

Colleen's case. That bothered me for a time, but I finally concluded that it didn't really make a difference. Right was right."

*   *   *

Swanson's last eight months at the company were spent putting an end to his life in Midland and his career at Dow Corning. To leave this insular world behind them, the Swansons purchased a modest, but comfortable, home in Bloomington, Indiana. Both he and Colleen wanted to move south and they had initially looked at Indianapolis where they already had friends. But Bloomington seemed more welcoming. The community had the size and ambience that seemed to suit both of them. Several professors at Indiana University's business school were familiar to him because they had attended a seminar on how to integrate the teaching of ethics into their own business courses. Swanson had helped to develop this program as co-chairman of the Business Ethics Advisory Council sponsored by Arthur Andersen and Company. The university already boasted its own ethics center, The Poynter Center, and the Association for Practical and Professional Ethics was also headquartered in Bloomington. For someone interested in the field of ethics, it seemed as good a place as any to begin a consulting business and do some part-time teaching.

The Swansons visited Bloomington in April and July and found a home that would at least serve as their getaway from Midland. All the pieces were falling together for Swanson to conclude his career, from his reevaluation of Dow Corning's ethics program to Colleen's resolution of her lawsuit against his company. In May 1993—three months before Swanson retired—she had settled her lawsuit with Dow Corning out of court for an undisclosed sum.

Swanson's final presentation as a Dow Corning manager was before a group of 40 executives at an area operating board meeting on August 13, 1993. Following more than six months of work, Swanson and the other four members of the Business

Conduct Committee had concluded that Dow Corning's code lacked full awareness and understanding by some of the company's employees. It also lacked what he called "proactive role-modelling" and support by the company's top management. The code was no longer well aligned with the company's vision, strategies, and milestones. It was not sufficiently understood, valued, and practiced by all employees.

Every executive at Swanson's presentation that August afternoon knew that the session had its roots in the failure of the company's program to uncover the latent concerns that erupted into the breast implant crisis. Yet Swanson knew that even suggesting a direct link between the need to reassess the entire ethics program and the implant debacle would alienate nearly everyone in the room. So Swanson did not connect the two. "Going through the reasoning that led to the recommendations to revamp the ethics program without reference to the implant scandal was for me an act of intellectual dishonesty," admits Swanson. "But I knew that interjecting my personal beliefs would only sink my credibility with this group."

Swanson moved through his presentation without even a mention of the crisis enveloping the company. The practice of ethics at Dow Corning, he said, was too centralized to be effective in the 1990s and beyond. Swanson had discovered that the ethics code couldn't have enough of an impact if just a handful of executives swooped down on various parts of the company in periodic audits that had, in fact, become more involved with educating employees than in uncovering potential ethics violations. Besides, the company had grown so large over the years that at best the conduct committee could reach little more than 10 percent of the employees every three years. It was no longer possible for the members of the committee to understand the operations and intricacies of Dow Corning's many subsidiaries all over the world. And what good were the so-called audits anyway? They had failed to turn up any problems with breast implants. Swanson had decided that the peer pressure in a room full of employees with a couple of business conduct members was hardly conducive to frank, candid discussions about ethics. How many would be willing to stand up before their colleagues and imperil their careers to allege a violation of the company's code? At best, you could make employees aware of the company's guidelines and then hope that a violation would be reported by one who took the code seriously.

Swanson urged the company to decentralize its efforts, making line managers accountable for conducting ethics reviews and bringing the code of business conduct to life. Rather than hold a few general sessions every two or three years, the idea would be to hold many group sessions on ethics far more frequently. Ethics, Swanson now believed, had to be a periodic but regular agenda item in staff meetings throughout the organization and at every level. All these activities would be overseen by area Business Conduct Committees, each with a communications and feedback channel that would allow any employee at any time to raise a concern about an ethical issue without fear of retribution. In essence, the company's area managers would "own" the ethics process for their geographic areas. Ethics needed to be ingrained into the Dow Corning culture in a more fundamental way than it ever had been. "Simply stated, we need a new process approach," Swanson told his colleagues. "One that enables us to fully understand, appreciate, practice, and capture through the business activities and daily decisions of all employees the positive values of good business ethics."

After Swanson's presentation, CEO Hazleton made a few gracious comments about him and his years of service at Dow Corning before handing him a final present: a pigskin briefcase full of golfballs and a cash award. That was his goodbye after nearly 30 years with the corporation. Given his decision to recuse himself and become a corporate dissident, Swanson had expected no such recognition. Later, Hazleton himself would perform Swanson's "exit interview," in which the executive would turn in his company keys, employee badge, and corporate credit card.

*   *   *

At the end of August, Swanson left Dow Corning for the last time, exiting through an underground tunnel into the bright sunshine of a Friday afternoon. It was the earliest possible date upon which he could retire and gain full benefits as a Dow Corning employee who was 57 years old, with 27 and a quarter years under his belt. Indeed, Swanson took a few days of vacation time so he wouldn't have to return to work the following Monday or Tuesday. He walked slowly from the large brooding presence of the corporate headquarters to his car, relieved that he would probably never have to enter the building again. It seemed ironic that after all those years of working for Dow Corning—despite his dedication over most of those years to shaping the company's values and its standards of ethical conduct—he felt that he had not really known the soul of the organization.

At 7 A.M. the following morning, a North American Van Lines truck pulled into the driveway of the condominium where the Swansons had lived for the past year. As they watched the movers open the huge doors and throw out the pads that would cover their furniture and other possessions, Swanson again felt relieved. The most stressful and painful year in their 20-year marriage, a year in which he had been uncomfortably isolated at work, a year in which he had lost some friends, a year in which he had almost lost his wife, was coming to an end.

John and Colleen stayed in Midland for one more night, guesting with friends, then left early Sunday morning—skipping breakfast so they would not have to prolong even for another hour their long-awaited exit. Colleen drove her 929 Mazda, while Swanson followed in his four-wheel-drive Mazda Navaho. They drove out of town on Eastman Avenue and had one last look at the home they had loved so much, the red brick colonial that backed the 14th hole of the Midland Country Club. "It was a pretty day," recalls Colleen. "The sun was shining. I was a little numb because I was still quite ill.

But I can't say I felt sad. It was a relief to put Midland behind us."

An hour or so outside of the world's silicone capital, they finally decided to stop for breakfast. "We didn't look back," says Swanson.

EPILOGUE

The Swansons could leave Midland, but they could not so easily walk away from their personal tragedy. Although the removal of the leaking implants has slowed the roller-coaster of her debilitated health, Colleen Swanson continues to have bouts of severe migraine headaches, joint pain in her hips and shoulders, lack of libido, memory loss, hair loss, and periodic nausea. She suffers from a variety of allergies and must endure painful injections two to three times monthly to ease the symptoms.

In late May 1994, she underwent surgery on her right shoulder to treat adhesive capsulitis, or frozen shoulder. The excruciating pain she endured has been relieved, but she has not regained the full use of her right arm despite several months of physical therapy. Her orthopedic surgeon, moreover, doubts that Colleen will ever have its full use again.

Her most persistent health problem, however, continues to be fatigue. She lacks the energy and stamina that she once had and that most women of her age take for granted. On days when she feels reasonably well, Colleen looks like any other attractive, healthy middle-aged woman you might see in a shopping mall. She's well put-together, in stylish yet conservative clothing with just the right bit of makeup. But when she goes shopping or visits her daughter Kathy, who now lives an hour's drive from Bloomington, she returns home exhausted. It sometimes takes her two to three days to recover. The result: Travel must be carefully planned, always with the availability of medical care in mind. She cannot work, even on a part-time basis, and she must limit most of her social and leisure activities.

For some time, Colleen has been concerned about the effect the silicone in her system may be having on her ability to think and remember. Prior to having implants, she was able to focus in and concentrate for extended periods on vast amounts of written material. Her comprehension and retention were excellent, according to John Swanson. But in recent years, both have slipped appreciably.

Soon after settling in Bloomington, Colleen and John began to interview doctors in the area who could treat her. They discovered Dr. Lois Lambrecht, an internist who had recently moved to Bloomington from Indianapolis. Dr. Lambrecht had some familiarity with silicone and its potential effects, but also read several medical journal articles on silicone cases supplied by the Swansons.

Colleen is impressed not only by the physician's willingness to learn more about silicone, but also by the care and support Dr. Lambrecht shows her patients. She has coached Colleen about her diet, about exercise, and about the importance of a holistic approach to regaining her health. Dr. Lambrecht has also been candid. "I have to tell you," she said to Colleen in early 1994, "right now there is no cure for what you have. But let's try a few things that can't hurt you and just may help you."

During the summer of 1994, Dr. Lambrecht suggested that Colleen try Pycnogenol, a natural product derived from the bark of the maritime pine tree. A powerful antioxidant, the substance has been researched and used extensively in Europe since the late 1960s, but was only recently introduced in the United States. Colleen's doctor believes that a daily dose of 50 milligrams might help counter some of her auto-immune-system problems. Colleen has taken Pycnogenol for more than a year and is convinced that it works for her.

Besides suffering from a host of symptoms that refuse to go away, she says she has been hurt by the loss of her good Dow Corning friends who refuse to acknowledge that some people can be harmed by silicone implants. When she makes new friends, Colleen usually avoids discussing her condition because she remains embarrassed to say that her health problems were caused by a cosmetic procedure.

But on one occasion, she decided to attend a support group for women with silicone breast implants in Indianapolis. About a dozen patients gathered for the session. They nearly gasped when Colleen revealed that her husband once worked for Dow Corning Corporation. She encouraged the group to focus first and foremost on getting better. "You have to believe you *will* improve and work at it every day," she told the Indianapolis group. "That is much more important than feeling bitterness toward the manufacturers or making a lawsuit the focal point of your existence."

Each day, Colleen still grapples with her own problems. "I don't think I've ever felt sorry for myself," she says. "I have a lot of days when I cry, but it's because of not being able to do things I would like to do. My fatigue is still bad, but now I can keep up the house and can go out more often. Still, this body is not very nice to look at. But John has never made me feel bad about how I look. All the discomfort I have with my appearance has been in my own mind. Someday, John may be ill, and I hope I'll be here to take care of him."

John Swanson, meantime, has spent much of his retirement thinking back on his career at Dow Corning and the company's implant crisis. He scans the newspapers daily for news about the crisis, ever in search of all the pieces to a mystifying puzzle that has now created headlines for four years. He has participated in lectures on business ethics before MBA students at Indiana University's School of Business—something he hopes to do more of in the future. And he has cooperated with several academic ethicists who have written case studies on Dow Corning and the implant controversy that are already being taught to MBA students at business schools. He plans to write extensively about the practice of business ethics in global organizations. "On a variety of issues other than implants," he adds.

A good deal of his time is spent nursing his wife back to health. "Through it all," he says, "Colleen certainly hasn't given up on herself. She desperately wants to get better. She energizes her spirit by bringing her special joy into the lives of her children, her grandchildren, and, not the least of all, me.

At her very lowest and sickest point, she was somehow always able to display her love and her caring nature. Short of death, we've been through the worst of times together and we are surviving. We now understand how shared tragedy can work to unite people who were already very close."

Swanson feels little sympathy for his former employer as an army of plaintiff attorneys, seeking to claim at least $1 billion of the $4.23 billion global settlement in fees for themselves, swarms around Dow Corning. Though he agrees that some jury awards in product liability cases are outrageous, Swanson views Dow Corning's legal woes as a "predictable outgrowth of its own consistent ineptitude" at managing the implant crisis. The legal assault, he argues, "is more of an effect rather than a primary cause of the company's fundamental troubles. The fact is, the company had numerous warnings and many opportunities from 1976 through the early 1990s to get out of the implant business gracefully. Instead, it chose a full speed ahead, damn the torpedoes approach that ultimately forced the parent companies to pull in the reins. In addition to the ethical issues involved, Dow Corning's failure to heed the many warning signals over the years was simply bad business judgment."

*   *   *

Like most of the women who have had serious concerns and complaints about their implants, Kathleen Anneken and Sybil Goldrich of Command Trust Network look forward to the day when they can put the controversy behind them. Anneken wants to clear her home of all the records and files from women with breast implants and get on with her life as soon as things calm down. Mostly, she'd like to paint again. The last time she put a brush to canvas was in 1988, when she sold landscapes through an interior designer. Since then, however, Command Trust has taken nearly all of her time.

Goldrich, who has been active in monitoring the negotiations for the global settlement fund, also hopes to call it quits after the settlement is completed. Recently, just before dying of cancer, Goldrich's mother urged her to move on. "Why don't you write a dirty novel and get rich?" Goldrich recalls her mother asking. "I said, 'I can't let go.' Once the deal is signed and complete, Kathleen and I will fold our tents and go away, sort of."

Dow Corning's bankruptcy filing disrupts those plans for now. "I look forward to being a trustee on the Dow Corning bankruptcy," says Goldrich. "That is my dream. That company belongs to the women because its executives relinquished their right to run it when they injured so many women and refused to take responsibility for it."

*   *   *

Goldrich may very well get her wish. On May 15, 1995, Dow Corning Corporation filed for federal bankruptcy protection in nearby Bay City, Michigan. For John Swanson and many other observers of the crisis, it was not an unexpected or shocking decision—it was the sorry conclusion to a management debacle. Overwhelmed by claims for damages from women with breast implants, Dow Corning is now battling litigants, lawyers, creditors, and its own insurers, who have refused to pay most of the claims.

Yet, momentum is swinging the company's way. The Justice Department had dropped a criminal investigation of the company due to insufficient evidence. In June 1993, Dow Corning won a highly publicized lawsuit brought against it by Tammy Turner McCartney, a topless dancer in Denver, who alleged that her implants caused her health problems. Several research studies from such prestigious institutions as Harvard University, the Mayo Clinic, Johns Hopkins, and the University of Michigan seem to support the company's position that women with implants are no more likely to contract disease than women without implants. And the British government has allowed silicone implants to remain on the market, concluding that women with implants face no greater risk of developing auto-immune disease than the general population.

Dow Corning, moreover, has assembled a high-powered legal team to help plot its strategy and defend it in the courts. Sheila Birnbaum of New York–based Skadden, Arps, Slate, Meagher and Flom is handling key legal issues in lawsuits across the country, as well as a multidistrict litigation concentrated in a United States District Court in Birmingham, Alabama. The so-called "Queen of Torts" and one of 100 of the most powerful lawyers in the country according to *The National Law Journal,* Birnbaum has helped companies fight product liability suits over asbestos, dioxin, lead paint, and DDT. David Bernick of Chicago-based Kirkland and Ellis is Dow Corning's national trial counsel. Frank Woodside of Cincinnati-based Dinsmore and Shohl is responsible for discovery and the depositions of experts.

None of this legal talent has come cheap. Dow Corning says it has spent $180 million in legal fees to this trio of law firms and the wider network of defense counsel it has established to defend itself in breast implant suits since January 1992.

Even the company's high-priced legal talent, however, could not prevent a bankruptcy filing after United States District Court Judge Sam C. Pointer, Jr., declared that the $4.23 billion global settlement was inadequately funded. Some 410,000 women with breast implants had filed claims under the settlement, which could be short some $3 billion or more. Dow Corning also faces between 5000 and 15,000 individual lawsuits from women who opted not to file claims under the global settlement. Judging by recent verdicts in these cases—a $5.2 million judgment in February 1995, against the company, among them—Dow Corning's future hardly seemed promising. In just 11 trials between January 1992 and July 1995, juries around the country awarded breast implant plaintiffs about $80.9 million in damages—most of them against Dow Corning's implant competitors.

Under pressure to cough up more cash for the settlement and to defend itself in nearly 200 individual cases before the end of 1995, Dow Corning decided to file for Chapter 11. The move effectively froze all the litigation against the company and also put the settlement in jeopardy. Dow Corning had pledged $2 billion to that plan over 30 years, with a $275 million installment due soon after the settlement was completed. But the company was getting little help from its insurance carriers, who also were embroiled in litigation with Dow Corning over the issue. Dow Corning said it had received less than $100 million of the more than $1.5 billion it believed its insurance carriers owed the company. "We don't have any more money to contribute (to the settlement)," insisted CEO Richard Hazleton. "It's not in anyone's best interest to bleed this company dry." The decision to file for bankruptcy was made shortly after the company reported that profits were up 33 percent in the first quarter of the year, to $49.5 million, on record sales of $612 million.

Dow Corning's Chapter 11 filing is one of the largest ever to result from product liability claims. Manville Corporation sought bankruptcy protection after thousands of plaintiffs sued the company because of asbestos-related illnesses and deaths. A.H. Robins filed for bankruptcy under a storm of claims involving the Dalkon Shield contraceptive device. In Robins's case, a $2.3 billion trust fund was put together in 1989 to settle nearly 200,000 injury claims filed by users of the contraceptive, which is believed to have caused pelvic infections and damage to the reproductive organs of women who used the product. The fund has since paid out some $1.35 billion in claims, and trustees estimate that all claimants will eventually be paid in full, with a significant surplus left over. It took Manville, however, six years of negotiations to emerge from bankruptcy court with a plan that gave asbestos claimants 80 percent of the company's stock. Indeed, the normal outcome of mass tort bankruptcies is that claimants eventually end up in control of the company.

The most immediate fallout from the Dow Corning bankruptcy hit the company's parents. Dow Chemical and Corning Incorporated both had to write off their $374 million investments in their joint venture as a result of the bankruptcy filing. Because Dow Chemical researchers helped in early safety studies of silicone and had once owned an Italian subsidiary that distributed implants abroad, a judge also ruled that Dow could be sued by plaintiffs for injuries and illnesses caused by breast implants.

Dow Corning's decision to file for bankruptcy was roundly chastised by breast-implant litigants, their lawyers, and other critics. Norman D. Anderson, a professor at Johns Hopkins University who once chaired the FDA's advisory panel on General and Plastic Surgery Devices, says the decision was typical "of a company that has consistently put its own survival ahead of ethical considerations." A long-time critic of silicone breast implants, Anderson disagreed with the company's claims that there is no evidence linking implants with autoimmune disease and accused Dow Corning of funding what he termed "selective and supportive research."

The bankruptcy maneuver appears to be part of a new defensive strategy by Dow Corning to sway public opinion to its side and position itself as a victim of greedy plantiffs' attorneys. Two days after the bankruptcy petition was filed, *The Wall Street Journal* ran an opinion piece by CEO Hazleton under the headline "The Tort Monster That Ate Dow Corning." In it, Hazleton argued that lawyers eager to snare fat fees for breast implant cases were attacking research that supported the company's case as tainted because it was funded with Dow Corning money. "They harass with threats of legal actions not only these institutions, but also scientific journals that dare to publish the research and individual researchers themselves," he wrote. "They advise their clients with implants not to participate in large-scale epidemiology studies because reassuring results might damage their legal case."

A few weeks earlier, the company ran full-page ads in 19 major newspapers across the country, under the headline: "Here's What Some People Don't Want You to Know About Breast Implants." The advertisements claimed that since 1992, "17 United States and international studies involving 121,700 women have consistently shown no link between breast implants and disease." The company provided a toll-free number for readers to request summaries of these research reports. But once again, Dow Corning was selectively quoting from the studies and declaring them to be much more favorable to the company's case than they often were.

The company said, for example, that the Mayo Clinic report on 749 women who had received implants from 1964 to 1991 and 1498 women without implants "found no association between breast implants and the connective-tissue diseases and other disorders that were studied." The Mayo study, however, was not based on evidence from doctors examining patients for connective-tissue disease. It was based on nurses' reviews of the medical charts of implant and nonimplant patients. Moreover, the 749 implanted women were followed for an average of 7.8 years. Many doctors, and even the Mayo Clinic researchers, contend that women with implants would have to be examined for at least 10 years before serious illnesses would be likely to appear. The study's authors themselves reported the research's considerable limitations which place Dow Corning's own conclusions about the report in question: "We had limited power to detect an increased risk of rare connective-tissue diseases such as systemic sclerosis," the Mayo Clinic reported. "Indeed, we calculated that it would require a sample of 62,000 women with implants and 124,000 women without implants followed for an average of 10 years each, for a doubling of the relative risk of this condition to be detected among women with implants, assuming that the annual incidence of systemic sclerosis is 1.6 cases per 1000 women. Our results, therefore, cannot be considered proof of the absence of an association between breast implants and connective-tissue disease." After the study was published in the *New England Journal of Medicine,* six doctors wrote to the journal to report that 257 surgical revisions were performed on the 749 women in the study, suggesting "an implant failure rate in excess of 30 percent." Yet another study, declared by Dow Corning and some journalists as the most definitive to date, also found no major connection between silicone implants and immune-system diseases. The research, published in June 1995, was performed by doctors at the Harvard

Medical School and the Brigham and Women's Hospital in Boston. Once again, Dow Corning was the beneficiary of a score of positive headlines and stories. One prominent journalist, science writer Gina Kolata of *The New York Times*, even proclaimed that the new report "is so compelling and its results so consistent with previous studies that some leading rheumatologists contend that the issue of whether implants cause these diseases can now be considered closed."

However, the study tracked only a limited sample of women with silicone breast implants: just 876 patients. If the Mayo Clinic's reservations about its study were applied to this latest research, it would have been clear that the sample size of the Harvard report was only 1.4 percent of what would be needed to detect immune-system illnesses. The upshot: the study's meager size makes its statistical significance far less certain and even doubtful. Indeed, some critics suggest that the study group was so small that it would not have found a link between cigarette smoking and cancer. Moreover, the study's authors excluded all women who developed diseases after May of 1990. Yet, they included women who had implants in place for as little as one month, even though it usually takes 8 to 15 years after implantation for symptoms of autoimmune disease to show up. Even worse, three of the study's authors were either personally receiving money from implant manufacturers or had agreed to act as a paid consultant for an implant maker while they were conducting the study. Dow Corning also contributed $7 million to Brigham and Women's Hospital while the study was in progress.

If all that wasn't enough to cast considerable doubt upon the study's conclusions, there also was the fact the Harvard study failed to report on implant ruptures, hardness of the breasts, deformities, chest and shoulder pains—all complications more clearly associated with silicone breast implants. Nonetheless, some journalists, eager to report a contrarian story, used the research to support the notion that Dow Corning is a victim of a legal system that is out of control.

*   *   *

On the morning of May 16, 1995, Silas A. Braley was sitting at his kitchen table with a cup of coffee and the local newspaper, *The Fresno Bee,* when he read that the product he helped Dow Corning create nearly 35 years earlier had caused the bankruptcy of the company. Now 78 years old and retired from Dow Corning for 18 years, Braley lives a quiet, anonymous life in California. He tends a small garden outside his home and he reads a lot.

A few weeks before the bankruptcy, Dow Corning had sent him and other retirees a letter indicating that the company was considering a Chapter 11 filing. So the news didn't completely shock him. Yet, as a kind of co-inventor of breast implants and a former company employee who helped to promote their use, the news leaves him saddened. "I am heartbroken about it," he says. "I think it's a terrible shame. It's a sad commentary on our legal system. Dow Corning is a victim of a situation generated by the lawyers."

He recalls seeing, even in his local newspaper, advertisements placed by trial attorneys seeking cases from women with implants. "These women have an unknown material in their bodies that is very convenient to blame for any problem they have," claims Braley. "And there's no good way to prove that it isn't the cause of their problems. We need the scientific studies. We need to prove these obscure diseases are not caused by silicone. In the long run, I think the truth will come out. It will be proven that there are no links between silicone and these health problems."

Braley is like most of the company's former executives in steadfastly standing by Dow Corning. "I can say, without any qualification, that never in my 30 years at Dow Corning did I ever know of anyone doing anything illegal, unethical, or immoral," he maintains. "If anything looks unethical or illegal, it was not deliberately done. I have always had a high sense of ethics myself, and I have always been proud of working for

Dow Corning, because it is one of the most ethical, public-minded companies I have ever heard of."

Braley has no regrets about playing a role in the development of implants or about helping to create the Center for Aid to Medical Research that provided silicone to doctors for medical purposes. "I remember at one time being very proud of the center," he says. "We were making a contribution to humanity. I find it very disturbing and very disheartening that these results could have come from such good intentions."

*   *   *

The news of Dow Corning's bankruptcy filing has Maria Stern and Mariann Hopkins, who won the two earliest lawsuits against the company after alleging that silicone caused auto-immune disease, stewing. "It infuriates me," says Hopkins, who now lives about 60 miles north of San Francisco. "What they have done is unconscionable. I know a lot of women who are still suffering from silicone implants, and a lot of women who will be hurt by Dow Corning's bankruptcy. And it's just beyond my belief to see them claim that their product caused no harm."

For Hopkins, the last six years have been stressful. Though her disease has been in remission a few times, she is still on strong medication to prevent further deterioration of her body. While she has regained much of the weight she lost, she must go to physical therapy three afternoons a week. She continues to have severe muscle spasms in her arms, hands, and neck. Her back and knees remain swollen. She has been in and out of the hospital many times. In fact, Hopkins had just checked out after a three-day stay on the very day that the Court of Appeals ruled in her favor against Dow Corning in August 1994. And in January 1995, when the United States Supreme Court turned down the company's request to hear the case, Hopkins was ill yet again with a flu or virus.

It wasn't until late May 1995, nearly six and one-half years after filing her lawsuit, that Hopkins finalized the papers and received all of her share of the award given to her by a jury in 1991. She planted a new garden in her backyard in the spring of 1995 and spends much of her spare time tending her orchids and vegetables. "At times, I hate to talk about this anymore," she says. "But I know this will be a part of me forever. I try to remember that there are still a lot of beautiful things in life. You have to learn to concentrate on them. I get that as much as I can from painting and from gardening."

Maria Stern, meanwhile, left California and resettled in Idaho, trying to start a new life away from the ordeal and the publicity. She has found herself criticized by some activists, including Sybil Goldrich, for accepting the Dow Corning settlement that allowed the company to seal the most damaging documents in the case for years. Stern says she feels much better, though she suffers from lupus and is still taking medication on a regular basis to deal with it. Unlike Hopkins, who was never able to return to work, Stern finally felt good enough to accept a part-time administrative job at a local law office in early May 1995. She had been employed there for less than a week when she stumbled upon a bit of news that shocked her. The day after Dow Corning declared bankruptcy, she discovered that her new employer was one of many law firms throughout the country retained by Dow Corning to defend it against breast implant litigation.

*   *   *

Nancy Hersh and Dan Bolton, the two California lawyers who did much of the early breakthrough work on breast implant cases, each represent more than 100 women who have either filed claims under the global settlement or are pursuing individual lawsuits against implant makers. Mark A. Kolka, the attorney in Bay City, Michigan, who handled Colleen Swanson's case, says he still represents about 25 other women in implant cases. In the big-stakes game of product liability suits, however, they are small players next to the more famous trial lawyers who have rushed in to play roles in the litigation. Some of these contingency-fee attorneys, such as Charles E. Houssiere and Joseph D. Jamail of Houston, claim to represent as many as 2000 to 3000 women with breast implant problems. "These cases have become an industry," sighs Hersh. "There are hundreds of lawyers involved, but I did a lot of it without much money or any kind of notoriety."

For his part, Kolka is sick of it all. He claims that the latest safety studies on silicone "are so flawed in their methodology and scope that they have minimal relevance to whether silicone causes disease. There is still no study that shows this stuff is safe, period." He calls Dow Corning's decision to seek bankruptcy protection little more than a ploy. "You have a viable and healthy company which has taken advantage of a legal system it claims not to like," argues Kolka. "All the global settlement did was to buy them more time. It's just a game. They can't win it, by the way, but it's just a game to them. I'm tired of it all. These days, it's nice when a traffic accident walks through the door."

*   *   *

Dr. James L. Baker, Jr., the Winter Park, Florida, plastic surgeon who installed silicone implants into Colleen Swanson's chest and the chests of 4000 other women, had the honor of standing before his peers in March 1995 as the newly elected president of the American Society for Aesthetic Plastic Surgery at the group's San Francisco convention. He remains convinced that silicone implants are safe and that the Food and Drug Administration acted irresponsibly in banning them. "You can't blame someone who is diagnosed with a crappy disease, like lupus or rheumatoid arthritis," he says. "No one knows what causes those diseases. There are no known causes. Yet, someone on television says your breast implants can cause it. What are you going to do? You always want to blame a problem on something. That's the American way. It's a normal phenomenon. The media first went crazy with it and drove everybody nuts. But now we have these big studies that are very significant from the Mayo Clinic and other places. The trial lawyers say they are worthless because they are funded by Dow Corning and in part by the plastic surgeons. We donated $5 million to this fund to do more research. We want answers. We didn't go into this business to make money and hurt people. We went into this business to help people. So my philosophy is that if the lawyers feel that way, if they think you can buy the Mayo Clinic and Harvard University, why don't they take some of the billions of dollars they have made and fund their own studies?"

Meantime, Baker's own business in breast implants filled with saline has returned to normal after a brief downturn in 1992, when the controversy exploded in the news media.

*   *   *

Keith R. McKennon, the former Dow Corning chairman who chose Hazleton to be his successor, is retired and living in Oregon. Larry Reed, the former Dow Corning CEO who was demoted by the board in 1992 when McKennon assumed his job, is retired and living in Midland, Michigan. J. Kermit Campbell, the one-time implant czar who recused Swanson, joined office furniture maker Herman Miller Incorporated in 1992 as chief executive. He resigned under pressure in July 1995. Robert T. Rylee II, who once headed Dow Corning's medical products business, is now on the boards of directors of several small medical device companies.

Rylee again finds himself on the hot seat. On July 26, 1995, Rep. James A. Traficant, Jr., (D-Ohio), and 14 other members of Congress urged United States Attorney General Janet Reno to open a criminal investigation into allegations that Rylee perjured himself before a House of Representatives committee in late 1990. Traficant made the charge after learning that a former Dow Corning medical director alleged that Rylee ordered the destruction of an internal analysis of implant complication rates. It was the same memo that landed on Swanson's desk on December 14, 1990, four days before Rylee testified under oath that silicone implants were safe and that Dow Corning did not withhold any reports or studies to the contrary.

Rylee, who lives in Memphis, Tennessee, denies the allegation. He is angry that product liability concerns have driven many major chemical companies out of the medical business. "DuPont got out of the business after we did and that created a major shock wave," he notes. "There are some very small spin-off companies trying to fill the void, but they don't have the size and the resources to develop these products. You're not going to see the DuPonts, Dows, Monsantos, or Union Carbides get back into this business for 10 or 15 years, if ever. Meanwhile, people who need these implants will suffer because of it."

Dan Hayes, the former CEO of the Dow Corning subsidiary that made the breast implants who was once a good friend of the Swansons, is also retired. When John Swanson saw Hayes on a golf course last winter in Destin, Florida, Hayes politely said hello and quickly went on his way. Time could not repair the long-time friendship torn apart by the crisis.

*   *   *

In Minneapolis, John Swanson's birthplace, MBA students crowd into a classroom at the University of St. Thomas to debate the ethical and moral dimensions of Dow Corning's silicone crisis. To prepare for this class on business ethics, they digest a pair of case studies that feature Swanson as a key protagonist in an unfolding drama. The professor in front of them, Kenneth Goodpaster, knows the story well.

In the 1980s, Goodpaster was the Harvard Business School teacher who traveled to Midland to interview Swanson and other Dow Corning managers for Harvard's flattering case studies on the company's code of ethics. He has since updated his earlier research with the latest developments to befall both

Dow Corning and John Swanson, a man Goodpaster has come to admire over the years.

It takes little time before the classroom discussion becomes both animated and provocative. The MBA students, largely part-timers who have already put in a full day's work at companies in the Minneapolis–St. Paul area, debate the failure of Dow Corning's ethics code to uncover the breast implant issue. They argue about whether there is such a thing as "an ethical point of no return" beyond which the company's managers failed to suspend the sale of a product for fear that to do so could create even bigger problems. They talk about the moral consequences of a legal system that allows important information for women to be hidden from the public by a court seal. And they discuss John Swanson and his personal dilemma in the case.

The MBA candidates view Swanson as a person who tried to be a loyal team player and who initially exercised some independent judgment by trying to get the Dow Corning board to temporarily suspend the manufacture and sale of breast implants until further study. When the students learn that Swanson's wife was one of many women who believed her illnesses were caused by silicone, they see the painful irony in John Swanson's position, and it leads them to be more empathetic toward him.

Yet, many of them wonder why it took Swanson so long to finally leave the company. They wonder why he waited until he could retire. "They see him making the right decision to leave," says Goodpaster, "but they think it took him a long time to do so. You might say that it takes some of the heroism out of it, but it also puts some of the humanity into it. John Swanson was one of the most loyal people I have ever known in terms of giving the company the benefit of the doubt. I explain to them that it would have been very out of character for John to simply walk away from this.

"You have to look at what he did at that company. John was a key cheerleader in a way: he got out there and helped articulate the company's positions and promoted its ethical integrity. I never saw him more animated than when I saw him make presentations to groups on the ethics program at Dow Corning. It was a source of tremendous pride to him. It was energizing to John Swanson. He was invested here at a level that was profound," says Goodpaster.

"Dow Corning was John Swanson's whole life in a lot of ways. Some people could read this case and say, 'Hey, wake up guy!' But the fair response is to put this into context, and you'll understand why he took the time he did to make the decision. He never claimed to be a hero. It's a story about a real human being who made an excruciatingly difficult decision. It's a personal tragedy for him and others, and it's a corporate tragedy, too."

AUTHOR'S NOTE

I had tried to reach John E. Swanson for days to no avail. He had not responded to any of my many messages. It's not an uncommon experience for a journalist working on a controversial story. Yet, I felt his cooperation was vital to the article I was then reporting for *Business Week* magazine. The article—published in March of 1992—was to explore why Dow Corning's highly regarded ethics program couldn't prevent a nightmare at the company. At the time, Dow Corning was making headlines that would make any executive cringe. The stories alleged that the company knowingly sold silicone breast implants that could cause a variety of ailments, from painful hardening of the breasts to immune-system diseases—charges Dow Corning vigorously denied.

I urgently wanted to speak to Swanson because he was largely the creator of the company's ethics system and had been deeply involved in it since its beginning in 1976. I had come across his name in the upbeat case studies on Dow Corning's ethics program written by a Harvard Business School professor for MBA students and executives. But Swanson had no intention of returning my calls. The reason he refused to call me back, I would later learn, was that he had removed himself from having anything to do with the crisis. He was at odds with the company's policies on breast implants, personally conflicted over the issue of how safe they were, and thought it would be unfair and unethical to talk to a reporter about it.

Nearly two years later, however, I received a surprise call from him. Journalism is a funny business. Whenever you work on a story, you tend to become obsessed and consumed by its

247

every detail. You hurriedly telephone and visit with as many sources as possible. You spend hours sorting through all your facts and interviews. And then you devote perhaps a couple of hours to frantically writing the story against a looming deadline. Once published, the article quickly fades from memory, because you're already at work on the next one and the one after that—especially if you cover as amorphous and broad a topic as management, as I do.

Caught up in the weekly grind of work and having interviewed hundreds of people since I initially tried to reach him, I couldn't remember that I had even phoned Swanson some 18 months earlier. So when he introduced himself, I failed to connect him directly to my story on Dow Corning's ethics program. Swanson was calling for some advice. He was, he explained, a former executive of Dow Corning who was interested in writing a book about the silicone breast implant controversy. Would I be interested in the project? Could I refer him to any editors at New York book publishing companies who might be interested?

It was not an unusual call. Having written business books for four different publishers in the past decade, I often receive calls from potential authors seeking advice and help. But I had no interest in a collaboration. So I referred Swanson to an editor I knew at McGraw-Hill. A couple of months later, the editor called me and enthusiastically thanked me for the referral. He described Swanson's unusual story as a touching and compelling drama. Would I like to take a look at it?

The material that so intrigued him immediately caught my attention as well. I flew to Bloomington, Indiana, where Swanson and his wife, Colleen, now live, and spent a long weekend chatting with both of them about their lives and their experiences of the past several years. Excited by the gripping nature of the story and their surprising candor in telling it, I returned to New York with great interest in some kind of project. Eventually, I asked if Swanson would be willing to allow me to be the sole author of a broader, more objective book that would explore the crisis from all viewpoints. More interested in getting a balanced and objective story out than putting his own spin on it, Swanson agreed. In exchange for his major commitment in time, McGraw-Hill is providing him with half of the book's royalties.

To tell the full story, I interviewed dozens of other observers and participants in the crisis, pored over the depositions of key witnesses, and examined hundreds of documents—many of them never before disclosed by the media— now piling up in the mounting litigation against the company. I wrote the story as I saw it, using the Swansons as the vehicle to bring an often complicated and painful topic to life. Given his huge presence in the book, I allowed Swanson to check the final manuscript for any errors or inaccuracies.

Dow Corning, unfortunately, declined to make any of its executives available for interviews. The day after I signed the contract to write the book, I called the company's vice-president and executive director of corporate communications, Barbara S. Carmichael, to let her know that I would be researching the silicone implant crisis for the purpose of writing a book that would center around John Swanson. I asked for interviews with most of the company's leading executives, from Chairman Richard Hazleton and President Gary Anderson to former CEO Keith McKennon, and former CEO and President Lawrence Reed. My request led to some discussion over the telephone with McKennon, who ultimately decided not to be interviewed for the book.

Even my efforts to interview Dan Hayes, the former CEO of the subsidiary that made the implants and once a good friend of the Swansons, proved futile. At one point in November, Carmichael informed me that Hayes had agreed to cooperate. Weeks later, I was told that Hayes wanted to have a meeting with me and one of Dow Corning's outside counsel to go over "ground rules." Finally, near the end of December, I was told by Carmichael that Hayes did not want to be interviewed. "He doesn't feel good about his relationship with John," said Carmichael. "He's very bitter and he doesn't feel anything productive can come from it. He's angry at John's general position on this."

A final effort to gain Dow Corning's cooperation was made

in early June, 1995, when I sent the company a letter asking more than 50 specific questions. At that time, I also asked again for access to several of the company's key executives. Once again, Dow Corning declined to answer a single question or to make available a single executive for an interview. In a letter dated June 30, Carmichael wrote that Swanson's participation in the book "precludes the possibility of a fair, accurate, and objective evaluation of this controversy. In fact, Mr. Swanson has told Dow Corning that he cannot write this book objectively and suggested in late 1993 that we consider paying him for the rights to his unpublished book. We declined this proposal, advising Mr. Swanson that such an action would be a serious violation of our corporate values and Code of Business Conduct."

Swanson adamantly denies that he ever made even the suggestion of such a proposal. Three months after Swanson retired from Dow Corning, he wrote Chief Executive Dick Hazleton to inform him of his plans to write a book and to ask if Hazleton and other key executives would agree to be interviewed. Over the next several weeks, Swanson had several conversations on the telephone with Hazleton in an unsuccessful attempt to convince him that the book would be more balanced if it included the company's point of view from its top decision makers. Swanson even offered to return to Midland to show Dow Corning's top executives the outline for his proposed book. Now, Swanson believes the company has either misinterpreted that offer or is deliberately using it to suggest that his silence could have been bought, a charge he maintains is untrue.

In any case, Swanson decided not to write the book. My involvement in it, he believed, would allow for a more objective and balanced portrait of the controversy. As I began to write the book, I made every effort to include Dow Corning's position on the issue of silicone breast implants by quoting from the company's official statements and documents and by using—where appropriate—comments by the company's executives from other public sources, including depositions filed in the multi-district litigation in Birmingham, Alabama. I also made numerous efforts to interview the company's former executives without Dow Corning's official involvement. Declining to be interviewed, former CEO Reed slammed the phone down after tersely declaring that he had no respect at all for John Swanson. Former Chairman Jack Ludington failed to return several calls made to his home. But some other former.executives were very helpful in providing details that add considerably to the narrative.

The result, I think, is a book that provides rare insight into the actions and mind of a sympathetic executive who found himself in moral disagreement with his employer. Swanson, moreover, was not just any other manager at Dow Corning. He was the long-time guardian of the company's ethics initiative, the person most responsible for making ethics a core value of the company. What makes his story all the more dramatic is the fact that the person he loves more than anyone else is central to the inner conflict he faced.

More than the personal story of an individual in moral conflict with the corporation, however, this is a case study of a company in crisis, under siege by angry customers, government regulators, and the media. Many aspects of the controversy touch on broader themes and issues. Among them: Are corporate ethics programs mere window dressing, or can they positively affect moral behavior inside a profit-seeking company? How does a corporation balance its reputation and financial well-being with the health of the users of its products? And when a public crisis hits, be it A. H. Robins's debacle with its Dalkon Shield birth control device or Exxon's disaster with the 00 oil spill, how open and candid should a company's executives be? What role should corporate lawyers and public relations consultants play in helping management deal with all the small and large decisions that need to be made in the midst of a litigation and media storm?

ACKNOWLEDGMENTS

The book in your hands would not have been possible if not for the candor of John and Colleen Swanson. I thank them both for their generous time and patience throughout the course of the project. David Conti, my editor at McGraw-Hill, has been an enthusiastic champion of this book. His insights and questions have made the final product far better than this author could have delivered on his own.

I also owe thanks to several of my colleagues at *Business Week* magazine. Denise Demong read through my draft manuscript with the attention to detail that she brings to any *Business Week* article. Steve Shepard, Mark Morrison, Sarah Bartlett, and Mark Vamos, my editors at *Business Week,* were gracious enough to allow me a leave of absence from the magazine.

Finally, my wife, Sharon, and my children, Jonathan, Kathryn, and Sarah, provided the support an author needs to get the job done. They understood that I needed to work intensely for long periods of time and that meant much time that might otherwise have been spent with them. I'm forever grateful for their understanding.

NOTES AND SOURCES

PROLOGUE

PAGE

1   *Precisely four weeks earlier:* Author's interviews with John and Colleen Swanson.

CHAPTER 1: CORPORATE RECUSAL

PAGE

5   *Everything he did that morning:* Author's interview with John Swanson.

5   *It meant that the 56-year-old manager:* Letter signed by M. E. Nelson, *Ms.*, January 1978, p. 7.

5   *As one Dow Corning executive calls him:* Author's interview with Barbara Carmichael.

7   *As the company's former chairman:* Dow Corning internal memo from Jack Ludington.

8   *Even the local newpaper:* Gordon C. Britton, "Dow Corning Learning All About Secrets," *Midland Daily News*, July 28, 1991.

8   *All this because of a product:* Author's interview with Keith McKennon for *Business Week* story.

9   *He had no knowledge:* Dow Corning memo dated March 31, 1977, from Chuck Leach to Bob LeVier. Dow Corning memo dated April 29, 1980, from Bob Schnabel to Milt Hinson.

9   *Nor had Swanson seen:* Letter dated September 23, 1981, from Dr. Charles A. Vinnick to Robert Rylee, president of Dow Corning Wright.

9   *And he was unaware:* Dow Corning memo dated June 24, 1991, from Dan Hayes on DCC Committee.

9   *Dow Corning would play down:* Company response from "Summary of Scientific Studies and Internal Company Documents Concerning Silicone Breast Implants," February 10, 1992.

11   *At first, she had suffered dreadul migraine:* Author's interview with Colleen Swanson.

12   *When Dow Corning's corporate medical director:* Dow Corning memo dated December 20, 1990, from Charles F. Dillon to John Swanson.

13   *He and his wife:* Author's interviews with John and Colleen Swanson.

14   *Campbell listened attentively:* Author's interview with J. Kermit Campbell.

16   *I very quickly understood his dilemma:* Ibid.

17   *Even though it is the largest:* Thomas M. Burton, "Implant Fund Too Small to Cover Claims," *The Wall Street Journal*, May 2, 1995, pp. A3, A12.

17   *Bankruptcy:* Milo Geyelin and Timothy D. Schellhardt, "Dow Corning Seeks Chapter 11 Shield, Clouding Status of Breast Implant Pact," *The Wall Street Journal*, May 16, 1995, pp. A3, A5.

CHAPTER 2: A COMPANY TOWN

PAGE

20   *The company has built:* "Small Town, Big Company," *Saturday Review*, July 10, 1965, p. 57.

20   *It's a clean town:* Author's interview with Nancy Britton.

21   *It's an atmosphere:* Author's interview with Gordon C. Britton.

22   *There was no more:* Author's interview with Arnold Zenker.

22   *Midland Daily News: Financial World* article by Adrienne Hardman.

22   *Midland's own agreed:* "Bleak town," *Midland Daily News*, January 1993.

24   *Dow Corning had the attitude:* Author's interview with Gordon Britton.

24   *Architects used:* "Company's HQ turned 25 in '92," *Midland Daily News,* April 22, 1993, Section D., p. 8.

24   *Colleen Swanson says:* Author's interview with Colleen Swanson.

29   *He arrived in 1966:* Author's interview with John Swanson.

36   *His program:* Author's interview with Laura Nash, an ethicist at Boston University's Institute for the Study of Economic Culture.

CHAPTER 3: SPARE PARTS FOR THE BODY

PAGE

39   *He was personable:* Author's interview with Eldon Frisch.

40   *In 1959:* Author's interview with Silas Braley.

40   *Try it in your animals:* Braley deposition, p. 38.

41   *Though the center helped:* Author's interview with Frisch.

42   *A doctor in Las Vegas:* "Escalation," *Newsweek,* October 25, 1963, p. 110.

42   *Complications due to injections:* Deborah Larned, "A Shot or Two or Three in the Breast," *Ms.,* September 1977, pp. 55–88.

42   *That's a creative act:* Al Reivert, "Doctor Jack Makes His Rounds," *Esquire,* May 1978, pp. 114–163.

42   *All told:* Statement of Dr. Norman Anderson before Human Resources and Intergovernmental Subcommittee of the Committee on Government Operations, House of Representatives, December 18, 1990, "Is the FDA Protecting Patients from the Dangers of Silicon Implants?"

43   *Another woman told* Ms. *magazine:* Ms., September 1977, pp. 55, 88.

44   *We went to New York:* Author's interview with Bob Emmons.

44   *If it caused no reaction:* Braley deposition, p. 73.

44   *In 1959, Frank J. Gerow:* Both Thomas D. Cronin and Frank J. Gerow are deceased.

45   *Gerow was working late:* Author's interview with Dr. James L. Baker, Jr.

45   *The implants:* "Hope for the Flat-Chested," *Science Digest,* December 1967, p. 69.

45   *Braley's Center for Aid to Medical Research:* Author's interview with Silas Braley.

46   *Eldon Frisch, who also worked:* Author's interview with Eldon Frisch.

46   *We talked:* Deposition of Silas Braley by attorney Mark Kolka in Fresno, California, dated April 23, 1993, pp. 109–116.

46   *Gerow spent an entire week:* Author's interview with Silas Braley.

46   *Braley informed Cronin:* Ibid., p. 118.

47   *Silicone was the only soft material:* Author's interview with Silas Braley.

47   *But when autopsies were done:* Author's interview with Marc A. Lappe, former professor of health policy and ethics at the University of Illinois College of Medicine.

47   *That looks and feels good:* Author's interview with Silas Braley.

48   *Gerow installed the first pair:* Ibid.

48   *We crossed our fingers:* Deposition of Silas Braley by attorney Mark Kolka in Fresno, California, dated April 23, 1993, p. 158.

49   *It had not been:* Braley deposition, pp. 109, 164–166.

49   *After he gave his paper:* Author's interview with Silas Braley.

49   *By 1967: Science Digest,* December 1967, p. 69.

50   *In a 1971 article in* Vogue: Simona Morini, "A New Aid to Plastic Surgery: Silicone, *Vogue,* March 15, 1971, p. 86.

54   *It's difficult to recall:* Author's interview with Colleen Swanson.

CHAPTER 4: SCULPTOR AND HIS CLAY

PAGE

58   *Swanson brought along the replacement:* Letter dated

February 4, 1974, from Dr. James L. Baker to Mrs. Colleen Swanson.

58   *She would like to be able to buy clothes:* Pre-operative report for Colleen Swanson from Drs. O'Malley, Douglas, Bartels, and Baker, P.A., in Orlando, Florida.

60   *He told me the procedure:* Author's interview with Colleen Swanson.

61   *"Cosmetic surgery":* Author's interview with Dr. James L. Baker.

62   Woman's *magazine:* Simona Morini, "Breast Sculpture, *Vogue,* January 15, 1971, p. 84.

62   *If plastic surgeons are the sculptors:* Susan S. Lichtendorf, "Are Your Breasts Too Small, Too Large?," *Harper's Bazaar,* September 1976, pp. 145, 174, 191.

62   *Just five months before:* James L. Baker, Irving S. Kolin, Edmund S. Bartlett, "Psychosexual Dynamics of Patients Undergoing Mammary Augmentation," *Plastic and Reconstructive Surgery,* 1974, Vol. 53, No. 6.

63   *Much to his amusement:* Ibid.

66   *Upward of a million Americans:* Diane K. Shah with Pamela Ellis and Ron LaBrecque, *Time,* October 23, 1978, p. 88.

69   *Baker, assisted by a nurse:* Operative report for Colleen Swanson dated 3/28/74 from Drs. O'Malley, Douglas, Bartels, and Baker, P.A., in Orlando, Florida.

CHAPTER 5: THE MARKET GROWS AND THE QUESTIONS BEGIN

PAGE

73   *Indeed, in one court battle:* Maria Stern vs. Dow Corning Corporation

74   *Within four days:* Dow Corning memo dated January 28, 1975, from A. E. Rathjen to mammary task force.

74   *We are concerned:* Dow Corning memo dated February 4, 1975, from T. Talcott and W. Larson to mammary task force.

75   *He was a bulldozer:* Author's interview with Tom Talcott.

75   *The time to act:* Dow Corning memo dated May 12, 1975, from A. Berg to mammary task force.

76   *He even suggested:* Dow Corning memo dated May 16, 1975, from Tom Salisbury to sales staff and other company officials.

76   *Still, by May 23:* Dow Corning memo dated May 23, 1975, from A. Berg to mammary task force.

76   *As the manufacturing plant geared up:* Dow Corning memo dated September 22, 1975, from J. Thompson to mammary task force.

76   *Soon, several salesmen:* Dow Corning memo dated March 2, 1978, from Frank Lewis to Milt Hinsch.

77   *Cran Caterer, a sales rep:* Dow Corning memo dated January 21, 1977, from Cran Caterer to John Woodard.

77   *In one instance:* Dow Corning memo dated April 29, 1980, from Bob Schnabel to Milt Hinson.

78   *Frank Gerow, who with Cronin:* Dow Corning memo dated December 12, 1975, from Tom Talcott.

78   *Ultimately, he quit:* Author's interview with Tom Talcott.

78   *Dan Hayes:* Tim Smart, "This Man Sounded the Silicone Alarm—in 1976," *Business Week*, January 27, 1992, p. 34.

79   *Dr. Donald Barker,:* Dow Corning memo dated March 19, 1976, from A. H. Rathjen to A. E. Bey, F. L. Dennett, R. L. Kelley, and W. D. Larson.

79   *I know:* Dow Corning memo dated March 31, 1977, from Chuck Leach to Bob LeVier.

80   *Still, the plastic surgeons:* Dow Corning memo detailing telephone call from Dr. A. B. Swanson to Eldon Frisch on March 16, 1977.

80   *Even Rathjen:* Dow Corning memo dated June 8, 1976, from A. H. Rathjen to A. E. Bey and C. W. Lentz.

81   *The first public hint:* Marjorie Nashner and Mimi White, "A 60% Complication Rate for an Operation You Don't Need," *Ms.*, September 1977, pp. 53–54, 84–85.

83   *While we truly believe:* *Ms.*, January 1978, pp. 4, 7.

85   *The culture had created:* Author's interview with Arnold Zenker.

87   *The response: Midland Daily News*, December 13, 1990.

CHAPTER 6: "WHY THE HELL ARE WE IN THIS BUSINESS ANYWAY?"

PAGE

93   *A once healthy woman:* Author's interview with Maria Stern.

93   *It wasn't long:* Author's interview with Mark A. Lappe.

94   *Swanson couldn't even recall:* Author's interview with John Swanson.

94   *Until then:* Author's interview with Nancy Hersh of Hersh and Hersh.

95   *Those cases:* Ibid.

95   *Stern went to Hersh:* Author's interview with Maria Stern.

95   *I went to five different doctors:* Ibid.

96   *Dan C. Bolton:* Author's interview with Dan C. Bolton.

97   *Indeed, the judge fined the company:* Memorandum Decision and Order of United States District Court, Northern District of California.

98   *I believe this proves the point:* Letter from Charles A. Vinnick to Robert Rylee, president, Dow Corning Wright, dated September 23, 1981, and released by Dow Corning Corporation.

99   *I feel that your company:* Letter from Charles A. Vinnick to Bruce Reuter of Dow Corning Wright, dated September 11, 1985, and released by Dow Corning Corporation.

100   *Sangster and Mannion:* Author's interview with Richard M. Sangster of Sangster and Mannion.

102   *Our engineers and scientists:* Author's interview with Bob Emmons.

102   *Some of the most riveting:* Author's interview with Mark A. Lappe.

102   *He was sent four boxes:* From a lecture given by Mark A. Lappe at a meeting of the Command Trust, 11/7/92, in Cleveland, Ohio.

102   *They [the brochures] were inaccurate,:* Ibid.

104   *Indeed, at one point:* Dow Corning's counsel Joyce Cram declined to comment on the case. David Lynch did not return numerous telephone calls to his office seeking comment.

105   *Dow Corning's lawyers:* Author's interview with Maria Stern.

105   *Why in the hell:* Author's interview with Robert Rylee.

CHAPTER 7: SILICONE CRITICS

PAGE

114   *Frustrated by her experiences:* Author's interview with Kathleen Anneken.

116   *Or so she thought:* Author's interview with Sybil Niden Goldrich.

117   *Nothing in my research:* Sybil Niden Goldrich, "Restora-tion Drama: A Cautionary Tale by a Woman Who Had Breast Implants After Mastectomy," *Ms.*, June 1988, pp. 20–22.

117   *Even so, her traumatic experience:* Testimony by Sybil Niden Goldrich before the Food and Drug Administra-tion's Medical Devices Advisory Committee, November 12, 1991.

119   *The issue was beginning:* James Rawley, "Dow Corning Corporation Scolded for Barring Implant Testimony," Associated Press, November 28, 1990.

120   *The Public Citizen lawsuit:* Ibid.

121   *Dr. James Baker:* Lorraine O'Connell, "Breast Implant Report Spurs Calls to Area Doctors," *Orlando Sentinel Tribune*, December 25, 1990, p. E7.

CHAPTER 8: AN ETHICAL ISSUE

PAGE

125   *Just five days before:* Memo from Charles F. Dillon to John Swanson dated December 20, 1990.

132   *It was an especially sensitive issue:* Dow Corning memo dated August 20, 1990, from Mary Ann Woodbury, regarding comments by Roscoe Moore, chief of the FDA's epide-miological branch, devices. Cited in Dillon deposition.

132   *She just said:* Charles F. Dillon deposition taken on March 18, 1994, pp. 141–142.

133   *We were all:* Dillon deposition, p. 164.

133   *Just four days later:* Testimony of Robert T. Rylee II before the House Subcommittee on Human Resources and Inter-governmental Relations, December 18, 1990.

136   *He does believe:* Dow Corning memo dated January 14, 1991, from Dick Hazleton and Jere Marciniak to Dillon, Rylee, Thiess, and Woodbury.

137   *He in turn will document:* Ibid.

137   *The studies:* Dillon deposition, p. 181.

Chapter 9: Taking Time Out

Page

149   *The issue of cover-up:* Memo from Dan Hayes on DCC Committee dated June 24, 1991.

150   *Kathleeen Anneken:* Author's interview with Colleen Swanson.

150   *Feng, a diminutive, Chinese-born plastic surgeon:* Author's interview with Kathleen Anneken.

150   *She had come:* Author's interview with Dr. Lu-Jean Feng.

151   *She impressed him:* Author's interview with Dr. William Shaw.

153   *She was objective:* Author's interview with Dr. Shaw.

155   *Guyuron concedes:* Author's interview with Dr. Bahman Guyuron.

155   *She found herself:* Dr. Norman Cole did not return several phone calls seeking his comment.

Chapter 10: The Little Candy Store Across the Street Gets a New Boss

Page

165   *The doctor did tell me:* Author's interview with Mariann Hopkins.

166   *I believed:* Tori Minton, "Implant Victim Started a Movement," *San Francisco Chronicle,* July 24, 1992, p. E3.

167   *You weren't going to find:* Author's interview with Dan C. Bolton.

168   *Even though Dan told me:* Hopkins.

169   *The jury felt sorry for her:* Former Dow Corning executive who requested anonymity.

169   *This jury verdict:* Dow Corning media release.

170   *If anything:* Author's interview with John Swanson.

170   *Robert Grupp:* Seth Rosenfeld, "Internal Reports Suggest Dow Corning Knew Silicone Could Affect Immune System," *San Francisco Examiner,* January 19, 1992, p. 1.

172   *How do you compete:* Author's interview with Arnold Zenker.

175   *One Texas law firm:* "The American Disease," *The Wall Street Journal,* January 20, 1992.

175   *It was sound-bite hell:* Author's interview with Barbara Carmichael.

175   *Anderson personally delivered:* Michael Castleman, California lawyer, "The Enemy Within," March 1993, p. 106.

176   *LeVier would dismiss:* Seth Rosenfeld, "Internal Reports Suggest Dow Corning Knew Silicone Could Affect Immune System," *San Francisco Examiner,* January 19, 1992, p. 1.

177   *Other studies:* Ibid.

178   *Indeed, when the FDA:* Christopher Drew and Michael Tackett, "Vicious Battle to Keep Silicone Implants Legal," *Chicago Tribune,* January 3, 1993.

181   *On the advice:* Doug Henze, "Dad's Advice Led to Midland," *Midland Daily News,* April 22, 1993, p. 5.

181   *But he made an unusual detour:* Ibid.

182   *McKennon didn't decline:* Deposition of Keith R. McKennon, taken on August 30–31, 1994, p. 137.

183   *When the safety of implants:* Elizabeth S. Kiesche, "Popoff on Implants and the Industry," *Chemical Week,* April 15, 1992, p. 8.

Chapter 11: Sell the Sucker

Page

193   *Campbell, however:* Author's interview with Campbell.

195   *While in Washington:* Author's interview with Sybil Goldrich.

196   *And I believed:* Deposition of Keith McKennon, p. 149.

Chapter 12: A Final Assignment

Page

212   *A Chicago native, Hazelton:* Kathleen Kerwin, with Linda Himelstein, "On the Firing Line at Dow Corning," *Business Week*, May 29, 1995, p. 37.

212   *Swanson had watched:* Author's interview with John Swanson.

212   *Discussing the failure of the ethics program:* Memo written by John Swanson to Richard A. Hazleton, "Some Thoughts About Business Ethics," dated January 17, 1993.

215   *Colleen's final year in Midland:* Author's interview with Colleen Swanson.

219   *And even Dow Corning:* Dow Corning internal Update newsletter to employees dated March 25, 1993, "Immunology Studies on Silicone Gel Completed."

219   *It clearly raises my concern:* Doug Henze, "Dow Corning Reveals: Study Shows Possible Immune System Link,' *Midland Daily News*, March 19, 1993, pp. A1–A2.

225   *Swanson urge the company:* Swanson's overheads and notes, "Code of Business Conduct, 1993 Revision."

Epilogue

Page

229   *Although the removal:* Author's interviews with John and Colleen Swanson.

232   *Like most of the women:* Author's interviews with Kathleen Anneken and Sybil Goldrich of the Command Trust Network.

234   *Dow Corning, moreover:* Author's interview with Sheila Birnbaum of Skadden, Arps, Slate, Meagher, and Flom.

234   *None of this legal talent:* Author's interview with Mark Kolka.

234   *Some 410,000 women with breast implants:* Author's interview with John C. Coffee, Jr., professor and an authority on mass tort litigation at University of Columbia's law school.

234   *In just 11 trials:* David R. Olmos and Henry Weinstein, "Maker of Implants Seeks Bankruptcy," *The Los Angeles Times,* May 16, 1995, p. A12.

234   *Under pressure:* Dow Corning statement to the media, dated May 15, 1995.

235   *It's not in anyone's best interest:* Kathleen Kerwin with Linda Himelstein, "On the Firing Line at Dow Corning," *Business Week,* May 29, 1995, p. 37.

235   *The fund has since:* Milo Geyelin and Timothy D. Schellhardt, "Dow Corning Seeks Chapter 11 Shield, Clouding Status of Breast-Implant Pact," *The Wall Street Journal,* May 15, 1995, pp. A3, A5.

235   *Indeed, the normal outcome:* Author's interview with John C. Coffee, Jr.

236   *Dow Corning's decision:* Richard Waters, "Dow Corning Files for Protection," *The Financial Times of London,* May 16, 1995.

236   *Two days after: The Wall Street Journal,* May 17, 1995, p. A19.

237   *Our results: New England Journal of Medicine,* June 16, 1994.

238   *One prominent journalist:* Gina Kolata, "New Study Finds No Link Between Implants and Illness," *The New York Times,* June 22, 1995, p. A18.

238   *Moreover, the study's authors:* Testimony of Representative James A. Traficant, Jr., before the House Subcommittee on Human Resources and Intergovernment Relations, August 1, 1995.

238   *Even worse, three of the study's authors:* Thomas M. Burton, "Harvard Study Finds No Major Link Between

Implants and Immune Illnesses," *The Wall Street Journal*, June 22, 1995, p. B7.

239   *He tends a small garden:* Author's interview with Silas Braley.

240   *The news of Dow Corning:* Author's interviews with Maria Stern and Mariann Hopkins.

241   *Nancy Hersh and Dan Bolton:* Author's interviews with Dan C. Bolton and Nancy Hersh.

242   *Some of these contingency-fee attorneys:* Christopher Palmeri, "A Texas Gunslinger," *Forbes*, July 3, 1995, pp. 42–45.

242   *For his part:* Author's interview with Mark Kolka.

242   *He remains convinced:* Author's interview with Dr. James L. Baker, Jr.

243   *On July 26, 1995:* Testimony of Representative James A. Traficant, Jr., before the House Subcommittee on Human Resources and Intergovernmental Relations, August 1, 1995.

244   *Rylee, who lives in Memphis:* Author's interview with Robert T. Rylee II.

244   *When John Swanson saw Hayes:* Author's interview with John Swanson.

244   *He has since:* Author's interview with Professor Kenneth Goodpaster.

249   *At one point in November:* Author's discussions with Barbara S. Carmichael.

250   *Once again, Dow Corning declined:* Letter dated June 30, 1995.

250   *Swanson adamantly denies:* Author's interview with John Swanson.

INDEX

269

ABOUT THE AUTHOR

John A. Byrne is a senior writer for *Business Week*, where he spe-
cializes in management topics and writes many of the magazine's
cover stories. His first involvement with the subject of this book
came in 1992, when he investigated and wrote a *Business Week* article on why Dow Corning's highly regarded ethics program (headed
by John Swanson) had failed to avert the implant crisis. Byrne is the
author of five other books, including *The Whiz Kids, Odyssey* (coauthored with John Sculley), and *The Headhunters*. He holds a master's degree in journalism from the University of Missouri and a
B.A. in political science and English from William Paterson
College.